Designing Occupation-Centered Curricula and Instruction for Occupational Therapy Students

This essential resource provides educators with practical guidance to design and deliver occupation-centered education for occupational therapy students.

Based on the Subject-Centered Integrative Learning Model for Occupational Therapy (SCIL-OT), a robust guide for instructional design, the book can be used to create and implement a single assignment, an entire course, or a whole curriculum. Applicable across different countries or regions, readers will explore the educational foundations and elements of the SCIL-OT, and how they can be applied to both teaching and creating learning materials. Supported throughout with stories, examples, and sample activities, the book is aimed at the growing numbers of graduate students and educators who create or revise occupational therapy curricula, courses, and learning experiences across university- and practice-based learning situations.

The first book to offer occupational therapy educators with how-to guidance in occupation-centered curriculum and instructional development, it will be an essential resource for forming future practitioners who embody the distinct values of this important profession.

Barbara Hooper is Professor and Division Chief of the Occupational Therapy Doctorate Program at Duke University, Durham, NC, USA.

Matthew Molineux is a Professor of Occupational Therapy and the Deputy Head (Learning and Teaching) in the School of Allied Health, Sport and Social Work, Griffith University, Australia.

Wendy Wood is Professor Emerita and former Head of the Department of Occupational Therapy, Colorado State University, USA.

"Learning occupation is 'the meat of it' for learning and practicing as an occupational therapist: we can thank an occupational therapy student referenced in this text for this concise insight. The Subject-Centered Integrative Learning Model for Occupational Therapy (SCIL-OT) is such a clever strategy to alert educators, students, and public-policy people to 'the meat' of this profession. The focus on education in occupational therapy is long overdue to move beyond the challenges worldwide to communicate our professional identity. We can celebrate the three authors who are outstanding educators who have written and presented on occupational therapy education for years. With this full text on the SCIL-OT, readers will see how, when, where, what, and why occupation differentiates our profession from others. I endorse the use of this model as a wonderfully efficient way to illustrate that 'occupation needs to become the central organizing framework for occupational therapy curricula', as the American occupational therapist Elizabeth Yerxa declared almost three decades ago. Learning occupation using the SCIL-OT will be a fascinating way for readers to focus the vast range of topics and experiences that underpin the seemingly ordinary yet incredibly complex learning in occupational therapy education. To me, learning occupation with the SCIL-OT puts occupation at the forefront in declaring clearly why the profession is named occupational therapy."

—**Elizabeth Townsend,** *PhD (Adult Education), FCAOT, Professor Emerita, Dalhousie University, Nova Scotia, Canada, Founding Faculty and second Director, School of Occupational Therapy*

"This book powerfully reaffirms the central role of occupation: claiming it and emphasizing its capacity to heal individuals, communities, and society in dynamic and meaningful ways. A resource that can be embraced across occupational therapy assistant and occupational therapy educational programs is essential, not only for teaching that occupation is our distinct value, but also for demonstrating how its bold and authentic application is vital to sustaining a healthy society. At a moment when the heart of occupation can feel lost and overshadowed amid discussions of models of care, this book brings it back into clear focus."

—**Arameh Anvarizadeh,** *Professor of Clinical Occupational Therapy, USC Mrs. T.H. Chan Division of Occupational Science and Occupational Therapy, Founding Member and former Chair of the Coalition of Occupational Therapy Advocates for Diversity (COTAD), AOTA Board President (2025–2028)*

"As the editor of the *Journal of Occupational Therapy Education* (JOTE), I have often been surprised how few articles submitted to JOTE explicitly include occupation, the cornerstone of our profession, as a key element. The Subject-Centered Integrative Learning Model for Occupational Therapy (SCIL-OT) was published in JOTE in 2020 and immediately filled this gap. The model is a roadmap to thoughtfully embedding occupation across the curriculum, so that it connects and guides all other content. This textbook expanding on the SCIL-OT Model is essential reading for all occupational therapy educators seeking to ensure their graduates truly understand how to engage in occupation-centered practice."

—**Dana Howell**, *Editor*, Journal of Occupational Therapy Education

"Congratulations to Dr. Hooper and her colleagues for this wonderful contribution to occupational therapy education. While the occupation-centered approach to curriculum is well known, this resource provides the 'secret decoder ring' of how to make it work in your academic setting. What a gift!"

—**Dr. Barbara A. Boyt Schell and Dr. John W. Schell,** *Schell Consulting*
Co-editors and Authors of Clinical and Professional Reasoning in Occupational Therapy

Designing Occupation-Centered Curricula and Instruction for Occupational Therapy Students

A Model and Practical Guide

BARBARA HOOPER,
MATTHEW MOLINEUX, AND
WENDY WOOD

Routledge
Taylor & Francis Group
LONDON AND NEW YORK

Designed cover image: Getty Images

First published 2026
by Routledge
4 Park Square, Milton Park, Abingdon, Oxon OX14 4RN

and by Routledge
605 Third Avenue, New York, NY 10158

Routledge is an imprint of the Taylor & Francis Group, an informa business

British Library Cataloguing-in-Publication Data
A catalogue record for this book is available from the British Library

ISBN: 978-1-041-06485-5 (hbk)
ISBN: 978-1-041-06484-8 (pbk)
ISBN: 978-1-003-63562-8 (ebk)

DOI: 10.4324/9781003635628

Typeset in Vectora LH
by Apex CoVantage, LLC

Dedication to Dr. Maralynne M. Mitcham—Friend, Mentor, Educator

Dr. Maralynne M. Mitcham was a pioneer who transformed occupational therapy education. She introduced distance learning in the 1990s and championed the profession's move to graduate education. She integrated research into teaching and advanced faculty development to meet new demands for learning design and assessment. Countless educators trace their growth to her mentorship. For nearly a decade, she partnered with the Center for Occupational Therapy Education, cheering on the ideas in this book and helping bring them to life through faculty development workshops. Her influence on occupational therapy education—and on us as colleagues and friends—is profound and enduring.

Contents

Figures

Tables

Acknowledgments

We thank our students and colleagues who have actively applied the Subject-Centered Integrative Learning Model to their teaching, learning, and curriculum design process. Their feedback and dialogue have advanced the model's development and offered encouragement about the model's promise.

Preface

Recently, an occupational therapy educator shared an experience that strikes us as commonplace in occupational therapy education. A student, entering their second year of the program, expressed relief and excitement that their cohort was finally "getting to the meat of it." After three semesters of studying occupation—how it functions as an agent of health, what happens when it is inaccessible, and how occupational therapists assess it—the cohort had entered a course that included instruction in a range of motion, muscle testing, sensory testing, and other assessments commonly emphasized in medical settings. "The meat of it," the student said.

The comment revealed how easily the core subject of occupational therapy—occupation—can be overshadowed by discrete skills and biomedical tools, even in programs that explicitly aim to be occupation-centered. It also reflected that new approaches to education are needed if education is to succeed in helping students gain a health perspective grounded in occupation.

More than 25 years ago, occupational therapy scholars and educators began using the sister phrases "occupation-centered practice" and "occupation-centered education." These phrases were coined not only to affirm the centrality of occupation but also to resist the drift toward body-function-focused interventions and curricula designed around discreet skills and subspecialties. They were a call to remember that the healing occupational therapists enable lies in connecting and reconnecting people to the occupations of life that give their days shape, flow, routine, and meaning.

In the decades since, our understanding of an occupational perspective has grown in depth and clarity. It is now widely recognized that engagement in occupation—by individuals, families, communities, and societies—is a source of health, wholeness, and healing. But it can also be a source of ill-health, fragmentation, and harm. Such is the complexity of the health-occupation dynamic.

Occupational therapy education must prepare students to understand and act on this dynamic. Through education, we raise up a workforce capable of seeing that many of the health problems facing people around the world stem from estrangement from occupations. That estrangement may result from health conditions, disabling environments, unjust laws, climate change, generational trauma, or habits formed around life-diminishing occupations.

This book introduces the *Subject-Centered Integrative Learning Model for Occupational Therapy (SCIL-OT)* as a framework for designing education. It supports educators in positioning occupation not as an adjacent concept, but as the core subject of learning—one that must be made visible, connected, and central across all levels of a curriculum. The model consists of five integrative elements: *occupation, topics, the knowledge community, the learning context,* and the *connecting lines* that link them. These elements guide educators to develop curricula and design learning that integrates all topics with occupation.

The SCIL-OT Model is not a prescription. It does not claim to solve every educational dilemma. Nor does it provide instruction in teaching methods or approaches such as team-based learning or constructivist approaches or teaching with AI. But it offers a new way of thinking about all methods and approaches—one that invites educators to design learning that is integrative, discipline-based, and deeply aligned with occupational therapy's distinct contribution to health and society.

Part I of this book introduces the SCIL-OT Model, tracing its development and theoretical foundations. It builds a case for why occupational therapy education benefits from a discipline-specific model and defines the key elements and principles of the SCIL-OT approach.

Part II brings the model to life, offering examples, design prompts, and strategies for applying it across four curriculum levels—the program level, the course level, the class session level, assessment, and practice education. Each chapter is written in the spirit of educational coaching—supporting readers to reflect, experiment, and adapt the model to their own teaching contexts.

This book is for new and experienced educators alike. It is also for graduate students anticipating their future in an educational role. It is for those who are ready to reimagine how we prepare students to carry forward the profession's distinct contribution to society—through education that is not only occupation-centered but also transformative and responsive to the evolving needs of communities and the profession itself.

Part I

The Subject-Centered Integrative Learning Model (SCIL-OT)

Need, Origins, Theoretical Foundations, and Overview

Part I establishes the significance of occupation-centered education to the profession of occupational therapy and to society as a whole. The Subject-Centered Integrative Learning Model is introduced as a guide for educators designing and implementing occupation-centered education.

DOI: 10.4324/9781003635628-1

Chapter 1

A New Model for Teaching Occupational Therapy's Distinct Value

INTRODUCTION

Designing Occupation-Centered Curricula and Instruction for Occupational Therapy Students is the culmination of decades of learning about how we, as educators, might most effectively design, implement, evaluate, and improve upon occupation-centered education. In writing this book, we imagined that many new and experienced educators (ourselves included) have learned from direct experience that realizing and strengthening occupation-centered education is challenging. We have learned that this work is neither prescriptive nor formulaic. It has no finish line nor endpoint. Instead, the work of designing, implementing, evaluating, and enhancing occupation-centered education is continuous, and is far more easily said than done.

In essence, occupation-centered education is the everyday work of educators who seek its realization and advancement. This work involves continually asking particular questions. For instance, we ask:

- How is the concept of occupation represented and manifested in our day-to-day teaching practices and across all levels of our curriculum?
- How might students develop deep understandings of occupation and its relationship to human health and well-being?
- How might students perceive that our program's occupation-centered vision, mission, philosophy, and learning outcomes are manifested in the designs of their courses, and why is this important?
- How might students draw meaningful connections between occupation and the myriad other topics they learn about in courses and through experiential learning?

We hold our answers to such questions lightly. With each new cohort of students (or new co-instructor, research opportunity, community partner, practice site,

DOI: 10.4324/9781003635628-2

and the like), we are called to rethink and refashion accordingly. In this regard, occupation-centered education offers us a continual wellspring for ongoing revitalization of ourselves as educators and of the curriculum in which our work is embedded.

Most formally defined, *occupation-centered education* refers to teaching and learning processes by which educators systematically link the concept of occupation to all aspects of a curriculum (Hooper et al., 2020). The aim of this book is to present the Subject-centered Integrative Learning-Occupational Therapy Model (SCIL-OT Model) with the hope that new and experienced educators alike may find this conceptual model a useful guide toward realizing occupation-centered education within and across multiple levels of their curricula.

In Chapter 1, we establish the need for a conceptual model specifically for occupational therapy education, and elucidate three basic premises upon which the SCIL-OT Model rests. These premises are as follows: (1) occupational therapy may be considered a professional discipline; (2) as a professional discipline, education in occupational therapy is, at its best, discipline-specific education; and (3) discipline-specific education centers around a core subject—occupation in the case of occupational therapy—and a related societal contract to uphold a particular public good. Lastly, we define and discuss the key terms in the name of the Subject-centered Integrative Learning Model.

OBJECTIVES

This chapter will help educators to:

1. Define and describe the nature of the work of occupation-centered education.
2. Understand the need for a conceptual model that offers guidance on the design, implementation, and evaluation of occupation-centered education across four component areas of a curriculum.
3. Understand the nature of occupational therapy as a professional discipline.
4. Define discipline-based education and situate it within a sociocultural view of professions.
5. Demonstrate the relevance of discipline-based education to occupational therapy education and the core subject of occupation.
6. Define and explain key terms in the model's name: subject-centered, integrative, and learning.

THE NEED FOR COMPREHENSIVE GUIDANCE ON OCCUPATION-CENTERED EDUCATION

By the mid-20th century, occupational therapy in the United States was characterized as being in a profound crisis (Kielhofner & Burke, 1980), even as having derailed (Shannon, 1977). This troubling state of the profession was attributed to its near-complete abandonment of the concept of occupation in both practice and education, as originally conceived by founders and early leaders such as William Dunton, Eleanor Clarke Slagle, Herbert Hall, and Adolph Meyer, among others. Hence, in the 1960s and 1970s, prominent scholars and leaders began to call for a renewed focus on the concept of occupation in educational curricula and standards (Fidler, 1966; Reilly, 1958, 1966, 1969). These calls led to important educational reforms, such as reestablishing the American Occupational Therapy Association (rather than the American Medical Association) as the profession's official accrediting body, and the return of humanities-based content (Presseller, 1984).

By the 1990s, renewed calls emerged from occupational science for what was first being called occupation-centered education (Wood et al., 2000; Yerxa, 1998). These scholars believed that re-centering learning from components of function to the core concept of occupation would require a curricular renaissance in occupational therapy education, essential to advancing the profession's distinct value, knowledge, and practice in the 21st century. This renewed movement toward occupation-centered education was also international in scope. Indeed, the 2002 accreditation standards of the World Federation of Occupational Therapists (WFOT) clearly supported the calls for occupation-centered education. The most recent WFOT standards require that, to be accredited by WFOT, all education programs in occupational therapy worldwide must include robust content on occupation (2026).

It is notable that the WFOT education standards (2026) offer general guidance on curriculum design. While instructive and helpful, WFOT's general advice falls short, in our estimation, of providing specific guidance on how educators might best connect all levels of the curriculum design to occupation and help students connect all the content they learn to occupation—the aims of occupation-centered education. Indeed, prior to the publication of the SCIL-OT Model in 2020 (Hooper, Molineux & Wood), no conceptual model existed that focused specifically on how educators might design, deliver, and evaluate occupation-centered education. We propose, therefore, that specific theoretical and practical guidance is greatly needed.

Such guidance is predicated on particular understandings of what constitutes a curriculum. Influenced by Lattuca and Stark (2009), we regard a curriculum as a holistic academic plan, one that offers a comprehensive, integrative, and dynamic blueprint for learning, considering the coherence across multiple components simultaneously. In academic programs that lead to degrees in occupational therapy, we identify four curriculum components in which the work of occupation-centered education transpires and across which it threads. As shown in Figure 1.1, these components are as follows: (1) the overarching commitments of a program, (2) academic courses, (3) classroom instruction and processes, and (4) approaches and experiences related to practice education. We inclusively use the term "practice education" to encompass what is also called fieldwork education, placement, work-integrated learning, and practice-based learning in other contexts.

The work of occupation-centered education involves envisioning a program's most substantial or big-picture commitments, beliefs, and reasons for existence (Figure 1.1). Thus, educators are called to formulate their program's distinct overarching aim, vision, mission, and philosophy, as well as ultimate learning objectives that students are expected to master. All these elements, which

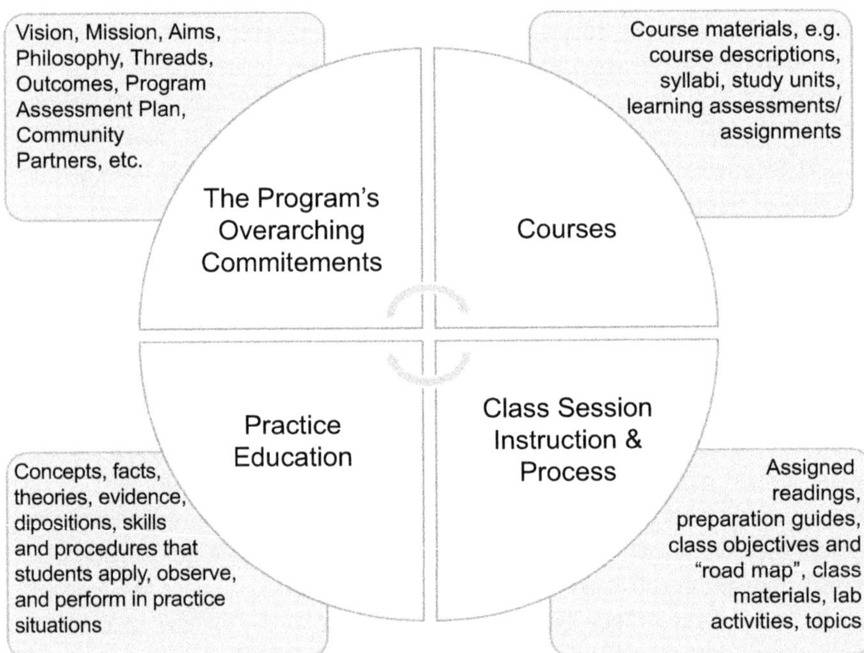

Figure 1.1 This book applies the Subject-Centered Integrative Learning Model to four components of an occupational therapy curriculum—the program level, course level, class session level, and practice education—and their associated elements.

often take the form of official documents or statements posted on websites and prepared for accreditors, are contextually situated. In other words, educators design these elements to be responsive to the prevailing professional, geographic, cultural, socio-economic, historic, and other contextual factors in which their programs are situated (Lattuca and Stark, 2009; WFOT, 2026). So situated, a contextually informed view of occupation can, and we would argue must, come into view at the program level.

Too often, however, particular conceptions of and commitments to occupation at the program component of a curriculum recede from view after they have been formulated. In other words, these elements are often only weakly manifested or "brought alive" in and across the other curriculum components of courses, classroom instruction, and practice education. In our experiences, formulating an occupation-centered perspective at the program level of a curriculum, while certainly requiring much thoughtful consideration and understandings of the contexts in which a program is situated, may actually constitute the easier tasks of occupation-centered education. For it is at the components of courses, classroom instruction, and practice education that occupation-centered education must be most fully operationalized and actualized for educators and students alike.

Guidance on occupation-centered education thus needs to be inclusive of all four curriculum components. Without such a comprehensive approach, research suggests that educators who are deeply committed to the concept of occupation may still inadvertently render it largely implicit (Krishnagiri et al., 2017). That is, educators may relegate occupation to the background, be that in how they design courses, lead classroom instruction and learning processes, or approach assessment.

This book, therefore, addresses educational approaches and teaching methods across all four curriculum components. *Educational approaches* refer to the "ends" and the "why" of teaching, the "broad theoretical and philosophical stances that encompass ideals about the nature of knowledge and content, educator-learner roles, why students learn and through what mechanisms" (Fenstermacher & Soltis, 2009, p. 7). *Teaching methods* refer to the "how of teaching" or specific instructional strategies that encompass "how learning is planned and organized, materials are created, techniques are executed, and learning is assessed" (Hooper et al., 2013, p. 10). It is important to note that no strict dichotomy exists between educational approaches and teaching methods. For example, problem-based learning (PBL) is perhaps most commonly thought of as a teaching method. Yet PBL also encompasses certain ideals about knowledge and how learning works, and so can also be seen as an educational approach.

Altogether, therefore, guidance on occupation-centered education should ideally support educators' understandings of *why* and *how* we explicitly center students' attention on the concept of occupation across multiple curriculum levels. The why of such guidance should provide sound educational theory for occupation-centered education; the how should encompass the activities of designing, implementing, evaluating, and improving a curriculum across its multiple levels. As next addressed, however, because no single source of theoretical and practical guidance on occupation-centered education exists, occupational therapy educators often turn to other resources for direction.

SOURCES TO WHICH WE TURN: CONTRIBUTIONS AND LIMITATIONS

In the absence of theoretical and practical resources on occupation-centered education, educators often turn to other sources. These sources include the following:

- How educators were themselves taught and what they were taught
- What has become an educator's beloved topic
- Published literature on occupation-centered education
- Accreditation standards and requirements
- Published literature on general educational theories and methods

Each of these sources offers important contributions and serves valuable purposes. Yet, either singly or collectively, they are piecemeal in nature when it comes to realizing and improving occupation-centered education.

Educators' Educational Experiences

It is common for academic and practice educators to draw on their own educational experiences as a foundation for teaching. These experiences can be valuable—especially when they exemplify effective instruction, deep learning, or transformative moments. Integrating such experiences into one's teaching repertoire can help educators connect authentically with students and model meaningful learning.

However, relying too heavily on personal experience can limit instructional range. For instance, an educator who was consistently affirmed by a former instructor may come to equate good teaching with creating positive affective experiences. While emotional safety and encouragement are important, basing one's entire instructional approach on affirmation risks overlooking the rigor, challenge, and complexity needed for deep learning.

Another concern arises when educators center their teaching around a single concept or topic they personally love. This passion can be infectious and engaging for students. Yet, when it dominates instruction regardless of course objectives, it can narrow students' exposure to the broader scope of the discipline. Students may leave the course with a deep understanding of one topic but without the integrative knowledge needed for competent practice.

Published Literature on Occupation-Centered Education

Of course, educators diligently gather and consult the relatively small number of published articles on occupation-centered education. Appendix A identifies some examples of this literature that we have variously found useful in our own educational practices or authored. Among other possible benefits, this literature can help educators understand why occupation-centered education is important. It can also help us elucidate our guiding philosophies and learning outcomes for a program-level component, particularly if used to stimulate discussion amongst educators. We may decide as well to assign some of this literature as required readings for the course-level component. Discussions of the readings may also make their way into classroom discussions at the classroom instruction component.

These are all important contributions that the published literature on occupation-centered education can make to educators. Yet even when considered collectively, this extant body of work does not elucidate *how* educators might help students engage in deep learning of the concept of occupation within and across all curricular components.

Accreditation Requirements and Standards

Educators are especially likely to turn to accreditation requirements and standards (herein called "standards") that prevail in different jurisdictions worldwide. Understandably, we are especially prone to consulting accreditation standards when engaged in designing or redesigning curricula, or when seeking accreditation or reaccreditation of our academic programs. As important as they are, however, accreditation standards are not intended to guide the design, implementation, evaluation, or improvement of occupation-centered education. We therefore caution against using them as such for several reasons.

The purpose of accreditation standards is to help ensure that specific academic programs can provide evidence of having met all minimum criteria for accreditation. Hence, whether those of WFOT (2026), the Accreditation Council for Occupational Therapy Education (ACOTE) (2023) in the United States, the Health and Care Professions Council (2023) in the United Kingdom, the Occupational Therapy Council (2018) in Australia, or some other jurisdiction, accreditation requirements define a host of *minimally acceptable* criteria against which academic programs are judged. Requiring this evidence can be critically important in helping to maintain the integrity of occupational therapy education and, thereby, the integrity of the profession. Occupational therapy educators around the world are thus ethically obligated to understand and help meet the accreditation standards that pertain to their particular curriculum.

Because accreditation standards define only minimum criteria for accreditation, however, they offer scant guidance on what constitutes and how to realize occupation-centered education across all curriculum components. Typically, only a comparatively small number of requirements address required minimum criteria related to the concept of occupation. Moreover, in the United Kingdom and Australia (and perhaps other jurisdictions as well), regulatory bodies establish accreditation standards that focus mainly on public safety. They do not necessarily address the concept of occupation, nor occupational therapy's ethos and distinctive philosophy in great depth.

Thus, it is erroneous to presume that any set of accreditation requirements provides adequate guidance on how to design and implement occupation-centered education.

Hence, we propose that the SCIL-OT Model can guide curricular development and revision work in a manner that aligns with accreditation standards while not being driven by them alone. We have found that first completed drafts of new or revised curricula already met most all accreditation requirements even though the SCIL-OT model first and foremost drove our curriculum work. We have also found that any outstanding requirements can be easily met by adding or modifying learning objectives, activities, and assessments within various courses or classroom processes. Moreover, curricula designed in this manner can, we believe, be especially innovative, reflective of a program's and students' contexts, and comprehensively occupation-centered.

General Educational Theories and Methods

As educators, we also commonly turn for guidance to general educational theories, knowledge about how people learn, and established pedagogical approaches that have emerged from the field of education. We perhaps especially turn to these resources when creating or revising courses, planning to teach individual class sessions, or providing practice education. Indeed, for over a century, occupational therapy educators, as well as educators across many professional disciplines, have benefitted from knowledge of the conditions in which people learn and adopted related pedagogical approaches that scholars in the field of education have produced.

For example, the following principles and related practices are well established within education (Fink, 2013):

- *People learn best when they actively construct knowledge rather than passively receive it.* Hence, educators have students work in collaborative groups and teams to explore and expand upon the boundaries of what they already know or believe.
- *People learn best when they can connect parts to wholes and situate what they are learning within a larger context that helps to clarify why what they are learning matters, rather than when they are presented with bits and pieces of information.* Hence, educators infuse their classes with client scenarios and stories to help students capture the bigger picture for learning discrete topics.
- *People learn best in authentic contexts rather than in contexts removed from real applications.* Hence, educators engage students in various forms of case-based, community-based, service-learning, and simulated practice experiences that immerse them in real-world complexities.
- *People learn best when they receive timely, clear, and honest feedback, rather than delayed, ambiguous, or insincere feedback.* Hence, educators structure learning to include accurate feedback early and often.

Additionally, scholars in the field of education have developed theoretical explanations for what constitutes learning under the above-described learning conditions. For example, learning occurs when:

- learning conditions raise student awareness of some of their taken-for-granted assumptions (transformational learning) (Mezirow, 2018).
- learning conditions help students continually draw connections among the discrete topics they are learning (integrative learning) and also among the big ideas of their field (idea-based learning); and help students actively assemble, evaluate, and justify knowledge for themselves (constructivism) (Bada & Olusegun, 2015).
- educators use authentic contexts that house the knowledge that students need to learn (situated cognition) and provide opportunities for students to transfer knowledge to and across multiple contexts (near and far transfer) (Battista, 2020).

Thus, a strong case can be made that the vast knowledge provided by education and learning scholars is indispensable to excellence in occupational therapy education. As addressed in Chapter 3, the SCIL-OT Model is accordingly informed by several of these theoretical understandings of how learning occurs. Educators in occupational therapy have, however, debated whether the rich body of knowledge from the field of education provides sufficient grounds for pursuing excellence in occupational therapy education (Hooper & Rodger, 2016). In light of our teaching experiences and curriculum work, we believe it is both necessary and insufficient. In other words, this body of knowledge can surely enhance occupational therapy education even as it falls far short of promoting excellence in occupation-centered education per se.

Stated otherwise, the benefits of educational theories, educational approaches, and teaching methods from the field of education expand considerably when we tailor them specifically to occupation-centered education. By careful tailoring, we transform "adopted" educational approaches and teaching methods into the means through which students learn the deepest tenets of occupation-centered practice of occupational therapy. When we tailor adopted educational theories, approaches, and methods such that they help students continuously connect their learning to the reason occupational therapy exists, we create bridges to occupation-centered education. Moreover, we propose that occupation-centered education can be an exemplar of discipline-based education.

PROFESSIONAL DISCIPLINES AND DISCIPLINE-BASED EDUCATION

Throughout this book, we refer to occupational therapy both as a professional discipline and, for simplicity's sake, as a profession. Regardless of which term is used, we understand occupational therapy to be a professional discipline comprising educators, administrators, scholars, researchers, students, and practitioners who all contribute to the maintenance and evolution of the field. Because occupational therapy education can be considered a professional discipline, claiming that its education is discipline-based education seems obvious and hardly in need of elaboration.

On closer examination, however, claims that education is specific to particular disciplines or professional disciplines require elaboration. Consider that much content and many topics that we teach in occupational therapy are also taught to students in other health professions, for example, client-centered or evidence-based practice, the concepts of therapeutic use of self or participation, ecological practice models, or research methods. Similarly, many teaching approaches that we use in occupational therapy are also used by educators in other health professions, for example, simulation, case- and problem-based learning, standardized patients, and service learning. Even individual accreditation standards that we must meet are not discipline-specific; for example, standards related to communication, research, and leadership are required across professional disciplines. Therefore, if some content, methods, and accreditation standards are shared with other fields, then we need to look further for what defines and describes discipline-based education.

Discipline-based education (DBE) refers to teaching and learning processes that are used in distinctive ways in a discipline. Being distinctive to a discipline does not mean that certain teaching and learning processes occur solely within one discipline. Rather, being distinctive to a discipline means that there is something characteristic about *how* a discipline configures teaching and learning processes to educate its particular learners. The term, discipline-based education, originally grew from science, technology, engineering, and mathematics, or the STEM disciplines, and referred to their characteristic educational approaches. Overall, discipline-based education implies that specific disciplines, and professional disciplines, have distinctive in-house teaching and learning practices, which their educators routinely use to educate future practitioners.

DBE is synonymous with the term, *signature pedagogy*, introduced by Shulman (2005) through a large-scale study of professional education. Signature pedagogy refers to forms of teaching and learning that are characteristic of a professional discipline—the fundamental ways novices in a practice field are instructed "to think, to perform, and to act with integrity" (Shulman, 2005, p. 52). Drawing on the work of Schulman, Schaber (2014) proposed that occupational therapy has three signature, or discipline-based, pedagogies: relational learning, affective learning, and highly contextualized active learning.

To further clarify discipline-based education, we turn to a sociocultural perspective of professions, in general, and occupational therapy, specifically.

A Sociocultural View of Professions

A sociocultural view of professions begins with the belief that individuals, groups, and societies have unmet potentials that they can fulfill when certain public goods are available and accessible (Sullivan, 1995). Public goods are complex and include things like equitable legal regulation and social justice, environmental safety, education, reliable information, work, and healthcare. Ideally, societies make such public goods accessible and available to all citizens. Western societies distribute these goods, in part, through professions. Professions exist to oversee and serve as guardians of particular public goods. Each public good addresses a practical need or problem that exists in society.

Guarding a public good is complex work. To succeed in this work, a profession must create an immense infrastructure that consists of, among other elements, standards, governing organizations, formal education programs, apprenticeships, licensure, and workplaces (Sullivan, 1995). Through such an infrastructure, a profession upholds its societal contract to take care of, develop, promote, protect, and equitably distribute to society the public good for which it is responsible. To ensure ongoing fidelity to its societal contract, a professional discipline prepares its members, through discipline-based education, in the

- values, beliefs, and actions associated with upholding the public good and making it available to all.
- ways of studying, speaking, and writing about the public good.
- professional infrastructure that supports working on behalf of the public good.
- expert practices that equitably distribute the public good to society.

A professional discipline further prepares its members to continuously critique, debate, and evolve the knowledge, values, practices, and the infrastructure itself to align with the shifting cultural contexts and on behalf of sustaining the public good for which the field is partial guardian.

As a profession carries out this complex work, the public good itself becomes a way of perceiving and understanding the larger society and the profession's role in it. For example, the public good provided by social work pertains to enhancing human well-being and helping people meet their basic and complex needs, particularly those who are vulnerable, oppressed, or who live in poverty (www.socialworkers.org). In contrast, the public good provided by physical therapy is to improve quality of life through prescribed exercises, hands-on care, and patient education (www.apta.org). In contrast to both social work and physical therapy, the public good provided by occupational therapy is to improve health and well-being through occupation, that is, to help people fulfill their potential by enabling optimal engagement in occupation as relevant to their contexts.

Students in social work, physical therapy, and occupational therapy may all study some of the same content areas (e.g., client-centered or evidence-based practice) and may also all be taught using similar instructional methods (e.g., PBL or case studies). Yet the educational experiences, and the ways in which they are prepared as new members of their respective professions, will differ in important discipline-specific ways. The root source of these important educational differences is each profession's distinct public good, societal contract, and the infrastructure that its members have built and continue to build and strengthen to uphold that contract. Accordingly, members internalize their particular profession as part of their identity. Addressing this internalization, Sullivan (1995) explained that "through the institutions of professional schools, apprenticeships, licensure, and a collegial workplace, a high level of formal education and craft skill has become embedded, as it were, in the practitioners" (p. 11).

Altogether, then, a sociocultural view of professions involves three broad constructs.

- Society contracts with professions to provide specific public goods that help individuals, communities, and society thrive and fulfill their potential.
- To uphold the contract, professions create knowledge and complex infrastructures and prepare members through education to competently and equitably distribute the public good and continuously improve the profession's ability to do so.
- In return, society allows professions autonomy in creating the infrastructure, self-governance, and self-critique that will ensure fidelity to distributing a public good.

Because society contracts with specific professional disciplines to provide distinctive public goods (first construct), learners are educated in a discipline-based manner to ensure that they uphold their profession's respective societal contract (second construct) and carry out their professional role in ways that advance the public good (third construct).

Discipline-based education accordingly immerses students in the following:

- The complexities of the public good that their particular profession is expected to help realize, the role that public good plays in society
- The levels of organization and infrastructure it takes to ensure this good is accessible and available to all
- What exactly constitutes expertise in their profession

Moreover, discipline-based education is important because it helps students "learn their way around a discipline" (Bransford et al., 2018, p. 139) and how to "do the discipline" (Wiggins & McTighe, 2011). Such learning helps to ensure that each new generation can contribute to society precisely what the profession exists to contribute in ever-evolving, and more just and equitable ways.

When students know their way around, when they embody and can 'do' a discipline, so to speak, then they are not simply performing the instrumental or technical aspects of the field. Nor are they simply learning preferred content within the discipline, as if the discipline were a mere container of content and skills rather than a dynamic, living entity.

Rather, students study the discipline itself.

Students immerse themselves in the discipline's history, structure, governance, values, perspectives, beliefs, behaviors, ways of knowing, skillful actions, and societal commitments. Education that helps students learn their way around all these elements of the profession promotes student knowledge and skill development in equal measure to student identity formation. Education for formation helps students embody the complex "analytical thinking, skillful practice, and wise judgement upon which the profession rests" (Sullivan, 2005, p. 195).

Discipline-Based Education in Occupational Therapy

As the above discussion suggests, discipline-based education in occupational therapy refers to in-depth knowledge of occupation and its relation to health and well-being, how knowledge of occupation is generated and structured, the situations occupation-based experts in the field are prepared to address, the logic and reasoning occupation-based experts use to address those situations, how experts know when a situation is resolved, and the field's challenges and gaps. Occupation and the relationship between occupation and health and well-being are the public good that the profession upholds and distributes within societies.

Discipline-based education in occupational therapy thus also means that occupation is not just another topic in a curriculum. Rather, occupation is the core of curriculum design and all teaching, learning, and assessment. Foregrounding occupation at the program level of a curriculum (e.g., vision, mission, program outcomes, learning philosophy) (Figure 1.1) highlights for students that occupation and its role in health and well-being will fundamentally inform their learning throughout their time in the program. With occupation at the core of all instructional approaches and teaching methods, students can best connect all topics in the curriculum to occupation and also be assessed on how well they make those connections. Continuously connecting learning to occupation is in essence continuously practicing the logic, perspectives, and societal purposes of the discipline. As students practice making connections to occupation, they gradually transform how they see situations and people, and how they understand their role in helping people and societies thrive. When occupation seeps into how students see and act, the profession of occupational therapy has, as Sullivan (2005) described, become embedded in its future practitioners.

THE NAME OF THE MODEL AND ITS EDUCATIONAL CONCEPTS

Each of the primary concepts of the SCIL-OT Model—*subject-centered, integrative, learning*—merits definitions and explanations. These terms have broad interdisciplinary support and are mutually co-defining, meaning explanations of one invariably invoke the other two. We begin with learning, arguably the most important concept of the SCIL-OT Model. We then elaborate on the two concepts that modify learning in the model's name, subject-centered and integrative.

Learning

In the SCIL-OT Model, learning involves both external and internal actions and processes. Students engage in learning by

(a) connecting the concept of occupation to themselves, other people, groups, and communities.
(b) linking occupation to various topics taught across the curriculum.
(c) justifying how these connections inform their professional decision-making.

This definition of learning is supported by interdisciplinary theory. For example, Illeris (2018) describes learning as a dynamic interaction between the learner and their social, cultural, and material environment (external), alongside the psychological processes of elaboration and acquisition (internal). These processes occur at the intersection of content, motivation, and social integration.

The SCIL-OT Model reflects Illeris's transactional view of learning and also embraces constructivist theory. In constructivism, learning is an active process through which students build upon—and move beyond—their current understandings. Transformation occurs as students select and interpret information, construct hypotheses, draw connections, and make and justify decisions (Bruner, 2018).

Such learning requires a cognitive structure that brings meaning, organization, and coherence to new knowledge. In the SCIL-OT, this structure is rooted in occupation, enabling students to integrate diverse content while maintaining a clear focus on how occupation supports health and well-being.

Subject-Centered

A particular field's biggest ideas comprise its most essential cognitive structure or schema (Hansen, 2011). A cognitive schema is a unit of knowledge that helps guide understanding, action, and the acquisition of new ideas. These big ideas or schema may also be understood as a field's *core subject* (Palmer, 2017). Core subjects reflect a profession's hallmark philosophy; central focus of inquiry, thought, and practice; and what holds the highest importance. As Palmer (2017) summarized, "[E]very discipline has a gestalt, an internal logic, [and] a patterned way of relating to the great [subject] at its core" (p. 125).

For example, "movement and movement-related function" is the core subject of physical therapy. "The study of humanness in the health circumstance" is the core subject of nursing. "Materials and their limits and potentials" is the core subject of engineering. Disability and the enabling-disabling process is the core subject of rehabilitation (Hooper et al., 2014a, p. 188). In contrast to these core subjects, *occupation*—humans' innate need and drive for occupation and occupation's capacity to form and transform people, their health and well-being, and environments, communities, and societies—*is the core subject of occupational therapy* and the core area of inquiry in occupational science (American Occupational Therapy Association, 2020; Fortune & Kennedy-Jones, 2014; Hooper & Wood, 2023; Townsend & Polatajko, 2013).

Understanding professions as concentrated around core subjects implies that professional education must likewise be concentrated around core subjects. Optimal professional education is consequently *subject-centered*, as is the learning that students undergo. Applied to occupational therapy education, the interdisciplinary concept of *subject-centered* refers to making *occupation* visible and accessible to learners across all curriculum levels and their elements (Figure 1.1). This visibility and accessibility pervade all courses, assessments, and learning activities, even when students are primarily learning about other topics.

Given that occupation is the core subject of occupational therapy, one might reasonably ask: Why not use "occupation-centered" in the model's name? Briefly answered, we use "subject-centered" because this term reflects the model's interdisciplinary influences, particularly, interdisciplinary views of professions. Furthermore, when we, as occupational therapy educators, effectively apply the concept of subject-centered to our students' learning of occupational therapy, we continuously render the profession's core subject of occupation visible and accessible to our students.

Integrative

The conceptualization of integrative learning in the SCIL-OT Model reflects other interdisciplinary influences. Integrative learning refers to

> *teaching and learning processes intentionally designed for connection-making among these phenomena: the perspective and habits of mind of the profession, abstract knowledge, responsible application of concrete skills, the subjective experiences and objective needs of service recipients, germane evidence, professional reasoning, relevant features of the practice situation, and the identity of the practitioner.*
>
> (Hooper et al., 2014b, p. 470)

As discussed in Chapter 3, integrative learning is promoted on the basis that solving complex problems requires the ability to connect seemingly disparate domains of knowledge and practice (Hooper et al., 2014b; Huber & Hutchings, 2004; Palmer et al., 2010). Students demonstrate integrative learning when they interconnect multiple domains of knowledge and experiences with the complex needs of the persons they serve.

Altogether, the model's name, *Subject-Centered Integrative Learning - Occupational Therapy*, foregrounds congruence with interdisciplinary understandings of optimal educational practices and points toward their applications in occupational therapy. Thus, as applied to occupational therapy, learning that is both subject-centered and integrative means that occupational therapy students are actively connecting their understandings of occupation across all courses, assessments, and learning activities. It means that students are making these connections even when learning activities that primarily address one of the myriad topics, other than occupation, that are taught in a curriculum. It means that students' learning is inherently social and constructive, as understandings of occupation emerge within and are contextualized by considerations of diverse persons, groups, knowledge communities, and situations and contexts. The SCIL-OT Model is, therefore, a tool educators can use to enact discipline-based education in occupational therapy.

SUMMARY AND CONCLUSION

In Chapter 1, we

- Defined and described occupation-centered education and highlighted the need for comprehensive guidance on this topic.

- Endorsed a view of a curriculum as a holistic academic plan, offering a comprehensive and dynamic blueprint for learning.
- Emphasized that comprehensive guidance on occupation-centered education must include educational approaches and teaching methods relevant to four curriculum levels: program, courses, classroom instruction, and practice education.
- Advocated for discipline-based education in occupational therapy that centers around the profession's core subject of occupation and its related distinctive societal contract.
- Introduced the SCIL-OT Model as one conceptual framework to guide occupation-centered education.

Hopefully, this chapter has laid a useful foundation for the ensuing chapters in Part I of *Designing Occupation-centered Curricula and Instruction for Occupational Therapy Students*.

Chapter 2 builds on the discussion of discipline-based education by focusing on occupational therapy's core subject of occupation. Specifically, Chapter 2 addresses the importance of helping students learn in an integrative fashion about both specific occupations and the dynamics of occupation that pertain to health and well-being. Chapter 3 explains the development of the SCIL-OT model and expands on the three educational theories that inform the SCIL-OT Model: idea-based learning, integrative learning, and transformative learning. Lastly, the fourth and final chapter in Part I of the book presents the SCIL-OT Model, including its five key elements and their guiding principles and rationales.

The chapters in Part II of the book apply the SCIL-OT Model in everyday educational practices. These chapters are organized around the five elements of the SCIL-OT model and their guiding principles. Numerous pragmatic strategies, examples, and tips are offered to help design, implement, evaluate, and refine occupation-centered education within and across all four curriculum levels.

Ultimately, we hope that educators who care deeply about advancing occupation-centered education worldwide will find this book and the SCIL-OT Model useful. We also hope that occupational therapy students fully grasp the distinct contribution and promise of occupational therapy. Most of all, we hope that students learn how to bring this promise fully alive in ways that the diverse individuals and groups they will one day serve as occupational therapy professionals find valuable.

REFERENCES

American Occupational Therapy Association. (2020). *Occupational Therapy Practice Framework: Domain and process* (4th ed.). Author.

Bada, S. O., & Olusegun, S. (2015). Constructivism learning theory: A paradigm for teaching and learning. *Journal of Research & Method in Education*, *5*(6), 66–70.

Battista, A. (2020). Situated learning theory in health professions education research: A scoping review. *Advances in Health Sciences Education*, *25*(2), 483–509. https://doi.org/10.1007/s10459-019-09900-w

Bransford, J. D., Brown, A. L., & Cocking, R. R. (2018). *How people learn II: Learners, contexts & cultures*. National Academy Press.

Bruner, J. (2018). Culture, mind, and education. In K. Illeris (Ed.), *Contemporary theories of learning* (pp. 159–168). Routledge.

Fenstermacher, G. D., & Soltis, J. F. (2009). *Approaches to teaching* (5th ed.). Teachers College Press.

Fidler, G. (1966). Learning as a growth process: A conceptual framework for professional education. *American Journal of Occupational Therapy*, *20*(1), 1–8.

Fink, L. D. (2013). *Creating significant learning experiences: An integrated approach to designing college courses*. John Wiley & Sons.

Fortune, T., & Kennedy-Jones, M. (2014). Occupation and its relationship with health and wellbeing: The threshold concept for occupational therapy. *Australian Occupational Therapy Journal*, *61*(5), 293–298.

Hansen, E. (2011). *Idea-based learning: A course design process to promote conceptual understanding*. Stylus Publishing.

Hooper, B., Krishnagiri, S., Price, M. P., Bilics, A. R., Taff, S. D., & Mitcham, M. D. (2014a). Value and challenges of research on health professions' core subjects in education. *Journal of Allied Health*, *43*(4), 187–193.

Hooper, B., Greene, D., & Sample, P. (2014b). Exploring features of integrative teaching through a microanalysis of connection-making processes in a health sciences curriculum. *Advances in Health Sciences Education*, *19*(4), 469–495. https://doi.org/10.1007/s10459-013-9481-5

Hooper, B., King, R., Wood, W., Bilics, A., & Gupta, J. (2013). An international systematic mapping review of educational approaches and teaching methods in occupational therapy education. *British Journal of Occupational Therapy*, *76*(1), 9–22. https://doi.org/10.4276/030802213X13576469254612

Hooper, B., Krishnagiri, S., & Price, P. (2020). The principles of occupation-centered education. In S. Taff, L. Grajo, & B. Hooper (Eds.), *Perspectives on occupational therapy education: Past, present, and future* (pp. 117–130). Slack.

Hooper, B., Molineux, M., & Wood, W. (2020). The Subject-centered Integrative Learning Model: A new model for teaching occupational therapy's distinct value. *Journal of Occupational Therapy Education, 4*(2). https://encompass.eku.edu/jote/vol4/iss2/1

Hooper, B., & Rodger, S. (2016). She said, she said: A conversation about growing education research in occupational therapy. *Open Journal of Occupational Therapy*, *4*(3). https://doi.org/10.15453/2168-6408.1307

Hooper, B., & Wood, W. (2023). A philosophy of occupational therapy: A framework for practice. In G. Gillen & C. Brown (Eds.), *Willard & Spackman's occupational therapy* (14th ed., pp. 38–53). Wolters Kluwer/LWW.

Huber, M., & Hutchings, P. (2004). *Integrative learning: Mapping the terrain*. Association of American Colleges and Universities.

Illeris, K. (2018). A comprehensive understanding of human learning. In *Contemporary theories of learning* (pp. 1–14). Routledge.

Kielhofner, G., & Burke, J. P. (1980). A model of human occupation, part 1. Conceptual framework and content. *American Journal of Occupational Therapy*, *34*(9), 572–581. https://doi.org/10.5014/ajot.34.9.572

Lattuca, L., & Stark, J. (2009). *Shaping the college curriculum: Academic plans in context* (2nd ed.). Josey-Bass.

Mezirow, J. (2018). Transformative learning theory. In K. Illeris (Ed.), *Contemporary theories of learning* (pp. 114–128). Routledge.

Palmer, P., Zajonc, A., & Scribner, M. (2010). *The heart of higher education: A call to renewal*. Josey-Bass.

Presseller, S. R. (1984). *Occupational therapy education: Yesterday, today, and tomorrow* (Order No. 8504293) [Doctoral dissertation, Duke University]. ProQuest Dissertations & Theses Global. https://www.proquest.com/dissertations-theses/occupational-therapy-education-yesterday-today/docview/303298478/se-2?accountid=10598

Reilly, M. (1958). An occupational therapy curriculum for 1965. *American Journal of Occupational Therapy*, *12*(6), 293–299.

Reilly, M. (1966). A psychiatric occupational therapy program as a teaching model. *American Journal of Occupational Therapy*, *20*(2), 61–67.

Reilly, M. (1969). The educational process. *American Journal of Occupational Therapy*, *23*(4), 299–307.

Schaber, P. (2014). Conference proceedings—Keynote address: Searching for and identifying signature pedagogies in occupational therapy education. *American Journal of Occupational Therapy*, *68*, S40–S44. https://doi.org/10.5014/ajot.2014.685S08

Shannon, P. D. (1977). The derailment of occupational therapy. *American Journal of Occupational Therapy, 31*(4), 229–234.

Shulman, L. S. (2005). Signature pedagogies in the professions. *Daedalus*, *134*(3), 52–59. http://www.jstor.org/stable/20027998

Sullivan, W. M. (2005). *Work and integrity: The crisis and promise of professionalism in America*. Jossey-Bass.

Sullivan, W. M., & Rosin, M. S. (2008). *A new agenda for higher education: Shaping the life of the mind for practice*. The Carnegie Foundation for the Advancement of Teaching.

Townsend, E. A., & Polatajko, H. J. (Eds.). (2013). *Enabling occupation II: Advancing an occupational therapy vision for health, well-being, & justice through occupation* (2nd ed.). CAOT Publications ACE.

Wiggins, G. P., & McTighe, J. (2011). The understanding by design guide to creating high-quality units. ASCD.

Wood, W., Nielson, C., Humphry, R., Coppola, S., Baranek, G., & Rourk, J. (2000). A curricular renaissance: Graduate education centered on occupation. *American Journal of Occupational Therapy*, *54*, 586–597. https://doi.org/10.5014/ajot.54.6.586

World Federation of Occupational Therapists. (2026). *Minimum standards for the education of occupational therapists*. Author.

Appendix A: Sample Publications Relevant to Occupation-Centered Education

Backman, C., Christiansen, C., Hooper, B., Pierce, D., & Price, M. (2021). Occupational science concepts essential to occupation-based practice: Development of expert consensus. *American Journal of Occupational Therapy*, *75*(6), 1–11. https://doi.org/10.5014/ajot.2021.049090

Bagatell, N., & Womack, J. L. (2016). Human capacity for action as core content in occupational science education. *Journal of Occupational Science*, *23*(4), 514–518. https://doi.org/10.1080/14427591.2016.1226682

Di Tommaso, A., Wicks, A., Scarvell, J., & Isbel, S. (2019). Uncovering educator perspectives of occupation-centred education in Australia: A qualitative study. *Australian Occupational Therapy Journal*, *66*(2), 174–182. https://doi.org/10.1111/1440-1630.12529

Hooper, B., Krishnagiri, S., Price, P., Taff, S. D., & Bilics, A. (2018). Curriculum-level strategies that U.S. occupational therapy programs use to address occupation: A qualitative study. *American Journal of Occupational Therapy*, *72*, 7201205040. https://doi.org/10.5014/ajot.2018.024190

Hooper, B., Krishnagiri, S., Price, P., Taff, S. D., & Bilics, A. (2019). A national survey of learning activities and instructional strategies used to teach occupation: Implications for signature pedagogies. *American Journal of Occupational Therapy*, *73*(5), 1–11. https://doi.org/10.5014/ajot.2019.032789

Hooper, B., Krishnagiri, S., Price, P., Taff, S. D., & Bilics, A. (2020). Assignment artifacts and what they reveal about how occupation is addressed in U.S. occupational therapy curricula. *American Journal of Occupational Therapy*, *74*(4), 1–11. https://doi.org/10.5014/ajot.2020.036012

Hooper, B., Krishnagiri, S., Taff, S. D., Price, P., & Bilics, A. (2016). Teaching knowledge generated through occupational science and teaching the science itself. *Journal of Occupational Science*, *23*(4), 525–531. https://doi.org/10.1080/14427591.2016.1238405

Hooper, B., Mitcham, M. D., Taff, S. D., Price, P., Krishnagiri, S., & Bilics, A. (2015). Energizing occupation as the center of teaching and learning. *American Journal of Occupational Therapy*, *69*, 1–5. https://doi.org/10.5014/ajot.2015.018242

Hooper, B., Molineux, M., & Wood, W. (2020). The Subject-centered Integrative Learning Model: A new model for teaching occupational therapy's distinct value. *Journal of Occupational Therapy Education*, *4*(2). https://doi.org/10.26681/jote.2020.040201

Krishnagiri, S., Hooper, B., Price, P., Taff, S. D., & Bilics, A. (2017). Explicit or hidden? Exploring how occupation is taught in occupational therapy curricula in the United States. *American Journal of Occupational Therapy*, *71*(2). https://doi.org/10.5014/ajot.2017.024174

Mernar, T., & Herzberger, L. (2025). Understanding accreditation requirement trends of teaching occupation in OT curricula. *American Journal of Occupational Therapy*, *79*(Supplement_2), 7911500178p1. https://doi.org/10.5014/ajot.2025.79S2-PO173

Palmer, P. (2017). *The courage to teach: Exploring the inner landscape of a teacher's life* (20th anniversary ed.). John Wiley & Sons.

Yerxa, E. J. (1998). Occupation: The keystone of a curriculum for a self-defined profession. *American Journal of Occupational Therapy*, *52*(5), 365–372. https://doi.org/10.5014/ajot.52.5.365

Zemke, R. (2016). Extending occupational science education. *Journal of Occupational Science*, *23*(4), 510–513. https://doi.org/10.1080/14427591.2016.1224010

Chapter 2

Teaching and Learning Centered on the Core Subject of Occupation

INTRODUCTION

As developed in Chapter 1, the concept of occupation is the core subject of occupational therapy because it captures the profession's unique perspective on humans and their health and well-being. The concept of occupation, therefore, lies at the very heart of occupation-centered education and, by extension, the SCIL-OT Model. The purpose of Chapter 2 is to introduce the SCIL-OT Model's *twofold perspective* on the core subject of occupation.

Consistent with discipline-based education in occupational therapy (i.e., occupation-centered education), we begin by proposing that students must learn what is distinctive about occupation as it is used by occupational therapists. For instance, students must explore questions such as:

- What is occupational therapy's distinctive public good?
- How are uses of occupation by occupational therapists different from uses of activity by members of other professions?
- How do occupational therapists apply occupation to meet the needs of an enormously diverse range of individuals, groups, and communities across a wide variety of settings?

This chapter introduces two dimensions of occupation that, when taught in tandem, can help students deeply 'get' occupation and appreciate the nuanced ways it is designed and delivered in practice. These dimensions are:

- *Specific occupations*
- *The dynamics of occupation*

DOI: 10.4324/9781003635628-3

When designing learning experiences from the perspective of the SCIL-OT Model, we propose that attention to both dimensions is essential. In relation to the dynamics of occupation, we also address a common challenge many educators face: how we keep advancing our own understanding of how occupation functions in relation to health and well-being, in order to teach students effectively about this complex relationship.

OBJECTIVES

This chapter will help educators to:

1. Discuss the implications of occupation as the core of occupational therapy for occupational therapy education.
2. Consider the impact of students' prior knowledge of and experience with occupational therapy on their expectations for learning.
3. Introduce two aspects of occupation deemed to be educationally vital in the SCIL-OT Model: specific occupations and the dynamics of occupation.
4. Introduce a self-assessment of educator knowledge related to occupation as the core subject of occupational therapy and occupation-centered education.

REFLECTIONS ON WHERE STUDENTS BEGIN OCCUPATION-CENTERED EDUCATION

In our experiences as educators, students often decide to pursue careers in occupational therapy due to inspiring encounters with occupational therapists. For instance, students frequently report favorable impressions of the profession after observing occupational therapists working with important people in their lives. Others describe being drawn in by seeing therapists do fun things with clients—like making a meal, molding a splint, or swinging on a bolster. Students are attracted by the variety of possible age groups with whom they can work. They are also attracted by the variety of work settings, including hospitals, schools, rehabilitation centers, hand therapy clinics, group homes, private practices, community centers, summer camps, and therapeutic riding centers or farms, among others. Although the specifics vary, students' decisions to pursue occupational therapy often stem from positive early encounters with the profession.

Students' original images and conceptions of occupational therapy hold great promise. At the same time, because much of the work occurs in the less observable process of therapist–client–environment interaction, these early conceptions are often underdeveloped or superficial. Some examples of beliefs formed from early experiences, as expressed by students in our classrooms, include the following:

- Believing that community programs without occupational therapists still provide occupational therapy because they are activity-based.
- Believing that having clients place small pegs in a pegboard, roll golf balls in a frying pan, squeeze therapy balls, use a sock aid, ride a scooter board, or stand up from a bed constitutes the use of occupation in occupational therapy.
- Believing that their previous roles (e.g., as nursing or rehabilitation assistants, activity directors, special education teachers, autism therapists, animal-assisted therapists, or therapeutic recreation specialists) were essentially the same as what occupational therapists do.
- Believing that physical agent modalities and exercises provided by an occupational therapist for injuries sustained as an athlete, musician, or dancer represents the essence of the profession.

These original conceptions shape students' expectations about what and how they will learn. For example, students who did not observe differentiations between occupational therapy and other health professions may expect their courses and labs to closely mirror those of students in other professional programs. Students who did not experience occupational therapists using or reasoning about occupation may expect a curriculum focused heavily on biomedical, sensory, or psychological treatments—mistakenly assuming that these treatments define occupational therapy. Students familiar only with medical settings may not anticipate, or even value, learning about occupational therapy in non-medical contexts.

In our experience, therefore, students often begin their formal education in occupational therapy with a mix of

- personally meaningful and compelling understandings of the profession and its concept of occupation.
- misconceptions and confusions about both.
- naïve expectations about what they will learn—especially regarding the focus on occupation versus the techniques or content they've previously observed.

As Ambrose et al. (2010) note, prior knowledge can both help and hinder learning in higher education. This is certainly true in occupational therapy education.

In this book, we propose that our role as educators is to guide students through transformational educational journeys—beginning on their first day and continuing through to their final day in our programs. Students' initial images and conceptions of occupational therapy are powerful catalysts for what they pay attention to and what they dismiss in our curricula. Early on, we can seek to understand and tap into what inspired them to pursue the profession. Throughout their studies, we can invite students to revisit, critically evaluate, and revise their original conceptions as needed. Most importantly, we can help them draw new and deeper connections to the concept of occupation.

As developed later in this book, educators can use *connection-making* to catalyze students' transformational journeys. By *connection-making*, we refer to teaching and learning processes that encourage students to draw increasingly informed, relevant, specific, and meaningful connections between the concept of occupation and the wide array of topics they encounter throughout their education. Through repeated and explicit connection-making—grounded in strong knowledge of occupation and related topics—students begin to discern how occupational therapy's skilled use of occupation differs substantively from the use of activities in other human services. These experiences also help shape students' professional identities as future providers and guardians of occupational therapy's distinct public good.

Of course, this is easier said than done. Occupational therapists and occupational scientists have spent decades exploring the links between occupation, health, and well-being—and there is still much to learn. Even without considering scholarship from other fields, a brief review of key textbooks and journals reveals the breadth and depth of existing knowledge. Given the complexity of the concept of occupation, how can educators help students graduate with a sophisticated, albeit entry-level, understanding of occupation and its relationship to health and well-being?

As developed next, the SCIL-OT Model proposes that educators focus on *two key aspects of occupation* in designing and delivering occupation-centered education:

- *Specific occupations*
- *The dynamics of occupation*

CENTERING TEACHING AND LEARNING AROUND OCCUPATION

Specific Occupations—Important but Insufficient

Specific occupations are perhaps the most easily understood aspect of occupation and would be readily recognized by all occupational therapists and occupational therapy educators. These are the distinct, concrete activities in which humans engage—such as dressing, cooking, playing with children, or feeding a pet. Daily lives—and entire lifetimes—are composed of a vast array of specific occupations. So numerous are these occupations that the profession has developed various taxonomies to categorize them, including:

- Self-care, productivity, and leisure (Polatajko et al., 2013)
- Activities of daily living, instrumental activities of daily living, rest and sleep, education, work, play, leisure, social participation, and health management (American Occupational Therapy Association, 2020)
- Self-maintenance, rest, leisure, productivity (Chapparo et al., 2017)

When we, as educators, help students understand these useful ways of categorizing what people do, we are teaching them about *specific occupations*. These categories are important because they provide insight into the potential purpose of an occupation. For example, based on a taxonomy, students may reasonably assume that showering—commonly classified as a self-care occupation—serves the purpose of maintaining personal hygiene and physical health.

We also teach about specific occupations when we use these classification systems to help students develop professional reasoning. For instance, educators may ask students to consider the four environments within the Canadian Model of Occupational Performance and Engagement (CMOP-E)—physical, social, cultural, and institutional—when analyzing occupational performance and engagement using the categories of occupations in the Canadian Model of Occupational Performance and Engagement, or CMOP-E (Polatajko et al., 2013). In this way, categorization supports students in being comprehensive when reasoning through the interactions of person, occupation, and environment.

Educators also deepen students' understanding of specific occupations by helping them recognize that, while useful, taxonomies offer incomplete insights into people's lived experiences of occupation. For example, students might initially assume that the purpose of showering is purely hygienic. But through dialogue and learning activities, they may come to see that showering can carry symbolic or emotional meaning. For one person, it might represent washing away the stress of the day; for another, a transition between school and home; and for someone else, a rare moment of solitude.

Not only can the meaning and purpose of a specific occupation vary widely between individuals, but it can also shift for the same person across different instances. Through these learning experiences, students begin to critically evaluate the tools used to understand specific occupations. They come to reasonably conclude that while categories are helpful, they are also limited—particularly in understanding the lived experience for a specific client (individual, group, community, or population) to engage in specific occupations, in a particular way, and within particular contexts.

Educators also teach about specific occupations when guiding students through occupation analysis—a foundational component of nearly all occupational therapy education programs. Common learning activities include having students engage in an occupation themselves or observe others engaging in an occupation and use structured tools to break the occupation into its component parts. One such tool is the *Occupational Therapy Practice Framework: Domain and Process* (OTPF; American Occupational Therapy Association, 2020). Students analyze specific occupations using OTPF domains such as contexts, performance patterns, performance skills, and client factors. Many of us—authors and readers alike—likely remember completing extensive analyses, sometimes ten or more pages long, of a single occupation during our own education.

Other common assignments may appear to go beyond teaching specific occupations, yet still maintain a strong focus on them. For example, in a time-use diary assignment, students identify their own specific occupations, categorize them using a published taxonomy, identify meanings, and calculate how much time they spend in different occupations or categories over a week compared, say, to a weekend. These assignments are effective for helping students observe how specific occupations unfold across the rhythms of their daily lives—whether during a weekday, weekend, or both.

The specific occupations we ask students to analyze are often shaped by the regional and cultural context of our programs. For instance, a program in a region with a predominantly young population may prioritize occupations common among children, youth, and their caregivers. A program aiming to prepare students to work with First Nations peoples may ensure that the occupational repertoire of local First Nations communities is meaningfully integrated into the curriculum. In this way, while all occupational therapy programs must ensure students understand specific occupations and their various classifications, the content can and should be tailored to prepare students for the practice contexts they are most likely to encounter. This approach also helps educators make thoughtful decisions about which occupations to include—and which to omit—when faced with a nearly limitless list of possibilities.

Teaching students about categorization heuristics, occupation and activity analysis, time use, and regionally relevant occupations is essential to occupation-centered education. However, even with this foundation, students may still struggle to grasp the full richness of human occupation, including for instance: the person as an occupational being; the emergence of occupation through interactions among environments and communities; the meanings and motivations individuals and groups ascribe to occupation; and especially how occupation actually works in relation to health and well-being.

To access these deeper understandings, students must begin to connect with the *dynamics that lie beneath specific occupations*.

Dynamics of Occupation—Linking Specific Occupations to the Complexity of Occupation and Health and Well-Being

The *dynamics of occupation* have been elucidated by occupational scientists and other researchers for several decades. Dynamics refer to the processes that both give rise to occupation and emerge from it, which has been the focus of occupational science since its inception. These dynamics encompass all the ways in which occupation serves as a primary source of health and well-being—and, at times, a source of poor health and ill-being. In other words, the dynamics of occupation represent everything we, as occupational therapists and scientists, articulate when asked: *Why do we focus on occupation? Why does occupation matter?*

It's important to note that each of the learning activities described earlier for teaching specific occupations can also support students in learning about the dynamics of occupation. However, doing so often requires one additional step—moving beyond categorization and analysis to interpretation and integration. For example:

- When students not only categorize occupations using a taxonomy but also portray how those areas interact to form a flexible occupational profile of a person, they begin to engage with the dynamics of occupation.
- When students analyze occupations across environmental, task, and personal domains—and then describe how the *transactions among those domains* shape unique occupational performance and experience—they begin to touch the dynamics of occupation.
- When students can explain to multiple stakeholders how a focus on occupation contributes to the health and well-being of individuals, families, and communities, they are beginning to understand the dynamics of occupation.
- When students observe and analyze occupational performance and also perceive a person's engagement as an expression of their innate occupational nature—a pull toward and from the environment—they are beginning to grasp the dynamics of occupation.

In this way, learning about specific occupations can serve as a portal into learning about the deeper dynamics of occupation. By distinguishing these two dimensions—*specific occupations* and *dynamics of occupation*—the SCIL-OT Model supports learning designs that move students beyond naming, categorizing, and analyzing occupations toward a more integrated and transactional understanding.

When considering the dynamics of occupation, we can identify *two key dimensions*:

- Multiple factors of occupational performance and engagement interact in multidirectional ways. These factors can both enable and hinder occupation, sometimes simultaneously. They include person, environment, and task factors, meaning, identity, temporal, and sociocultural factors, for example.
- The relationship between occupation and health and well-being.

To illustrate the first dimension, consider a simple example: a person is at home in the early evening with a cat meowing for food. The meows prompt the person to engage in the occupation of feeding the cat. A basic analysis might identify the environmental factor (the cat's meowing) and several person factors (sensorimotor and cognitive abilities) required to complete the tasks: moving to where the supplies are, picking up the bowl, opening the food packet, placing food in the bowl, judging the appropriate amount, and so on. Assuming the person has adequate abilities, these person factors enable occupational performance, and the occupation, in turn, draws upon and reinforces those capacities.

Yet behind this seemingly simple act lies a complex and dynamic interplay of factors. The occupation of feeding the cat arises from a web of transactions among less visible environmental and personal elements, such as:

- A sociocultural context that values cats as pets
- Systems for pet adoption or social networks that facilitate pet ownership
- A living situation that allows pets
- A physical environment that accommodates pet care
- Financial resources for food, healthcare, and pet sitting
- Transportation or social systems for accessing supplies
- Agricultural and manufacturing systems for producing and distributing pet food
- Regulatory systems ensuring food safety
- The person's history with pets
- The emotional meaning of the relationship with the cat
- The way pet care connects the person to others and to the community
- The influence of pet care on daily routines
- Expressions of love, care, play, and companionship

- Adaptations to life circumstances (e.g., pandemic-related isolation)
- The sensory experiences the cat introduces into the person's day and so on

For brevity, we've listed these elements. But to truly understand the dynamics of this occupation, students must create concept maps of how each one of these elements depends upon and supports all the others, especially how a change at any level impacts occupational performance and engagement throughout. Students must also describe how caring for a pet can directly relate to health and well-being, and how, therefore, health and well-being rely on the effective transactions of the whole system described earlier. Once students can make these connections, they begin to understand how the loss of occupation—such as no longer being able to care for a pet—can lead to a loss of health and well-being.

In sum, occupations arise in particular ways because of the transactional convergence of multiple micro- and macro-level environmental and personal factors. As an occupation emerges, it calls upon particular capacities—and the use of those capacities can, in turn, influence health and well-being, for better or worse. Occupational therapists become experts in enabling occupation, which is our profession's distinctive contribution to health and well-being.

The second aspect of the *dynamics of occupation* refers to the relationship between occupation—including all the complex mechanisms that give rise to, enable, or inhibit it—and *health and well-being*. As the previous example illustrated, understanding both the intricacies of occupation and its relationship to health and well-being is inherently complex (see Box 2.1).

BOX 2.1 OCCUPATION AS THE BASIS FOR SURVIVAL, HEALTH, AND WELL-BEING

The extent and quality of survival for individuals, families, communities, and societal and global populations depend on their health and physical, mental, and social well-being; health is the outcome of each organism having all essential sustenance and safety needs met and of having physical, mental, and social capacities maintained, developed, exercised, and in balance. This is achieved through what people do.

In turn, engagement in occupation depends on a level of health and its specific components, which are able to provide the energy, drive, and functional attributes necessary for engagement. In addition, survival as

> a health species depends on humans' capacity to live in harmony with others, and within an environment that can continue to provide basic requirements, ensure the continued acquisition of these requirements, and provided safety and education for the next generation (Wilcock & Hocking, 2024, p. 109).

While it may be tempting to shorthand this complexity with simplistic phrases such as "occupation is a mechanism of health" or "health through occupation," such simplifications must be used with care. They risk overlooking the multidirectional and nuanced transactions between person, environment, and occupation. As Yerxa (1988, p. 5) warned, oversimplification is "a hobgoblin for occupational therapy and practice"—and, we would add, for occupational therapy education as well.

Thus, our challenge as educators is twofold:

- To help students appreciate and explain the micro- and macro-level intricacies of occupation and its relationship to health and well-being
- To support students in applying this complex understanding to improve the health and well-being of individuals, communities, and populations

Occupation has been defined and explored extensively in the literature of occupational therapy and occupational science. A strong understanding of this literature can help students move beyond classifying and categorizing occupation and its related person and environment factors, toward a richer, more transactional understanding of how occupation relates to health and well-being. These insights highlight how occupation functions not just as a set of discrete tasks but as a complex, lived process that is deeply intertwined with meaning, context, identity, and health. One particularly useful synthesis comes from Molineux's (2009) review of literature published up to the early 21st century. These findings can help students move beyond surface-level classification and toward a more dynamic understanding of how occupation contributes to health and well-being.

- All occupations are active: they require physical and/or mental engagement. While the balance of these demands may vary, all occupations involve active participation by the person.
- All occupations have a purpose: while taxonomies (e.g., self-care, productivity, leisure) may suggest a general purpose, it is essential to understand purpose from the individual's perspective. Wilcock and Hocking (2024) further argued that occupations serve purposes not only for individuals but also for the human species.

- All occupations have meaning: this can be a contentious point, especially given the common use of the term *meaningful occupation*, which implies that some occupations lack meaning. In reality, all occupations carry some degree of meaning—though that meaning may be positive, negative, or complex. For example, cooking a meal to celebrate an anniversary may carry deep emotional meaning, while cleaning a toilet may carry limited or even negative meaning. Still, both have meaning. (See Molineux, 2009; Pierce, 2012; Polatajko et al., 2007.)
- All occupations are contextualized: they arise from and are shaped by specific configurations of context. At the same time, engaging in occupation can also influence and reshape those contexts, creating a two-way relationship.
- Occupation is a defining feature of being human: while this idea is debated, there is an implicit—and sometimes explicit—suggestion that the capacity to engage in and orchestrate occupations, and the intimate link between occupation and health, is central to what it means to be human.

Ultimately, we know students have begun to grasp the *dynamics of occupation* when they can explain, in specific terms, how occupation is the source of several pillars of health (Wilcock & Hocking, 2024). Some examples include the following:

- Fulfill basic survival needs (e.g., food, shelter, rest).
- Develop, use, and retain physical, mental, and social capacities.
- Generate income.
- Meet social needs.
- Meet learning needs.
- Live in safety and stable ecosystems.
- Contribute to and feel connected within families and communities.
- Adapt to environmental conditions and, in some cases, create environmental change.

HOW DO WE KNOW THAT WE KNOW ENOUGH ABOUT OCCUPATION AS EDUCATORS?

It is beyond the scope of this book to provide a comprehensive overview of the extensive literature in occupational therapy and occupational science that explores occupation and its relationship to health and well-being across individuals, groups, and communities. However, this chapter has highlighted the complexities of occupation, the nature of humans as occupational beings, and the multifaceted relationship between occupation and health and well-being.

The dual focus in teaching *specific occupations* and the *dynamics of occupation* means that we, as educators, must continue to develop our own understanding of occupation while also supporting students—recognizing that they cannot learn everything at once. Striking this balance is a central challenge in occupation-centered education.

OCCUPATION KNOWLEDGE SELF-ASSESSMENT

As we reflect on continuing to learn about occupation and its relationship to health and well-being, the following screening tool may serve as a useful starting point to identify individual strengths and growth areas for teaching the connections between occupation and health. The tool may also serve to screen program content strengths and gaps. Additionally, researchers have published a list of essential concepts from occupational science to support occupation-based practice (Backman et al., 2021). We have heard from several educators that the research has been useful as a tool in curricular review and teaching.

Instructions

Use the following screening tool (Table 2.1) to rate your knowledge in each content area below, with 1 indicating little to no exposure and 5 indicating extensive knowledge. After completing, review your scores. Use lower ratings to guide professional development such as a focused reading list, a journal or book club, a plan for selecting AOTA Inspire presentations, and other conference participation such as the Society for the Study of Occupation, the United States or International.

Table 2.1 Occupation knowledge self-assessment. Educators can use this screening tool to identify strengths and growth areas related to occupation-centered teaching and learning.

Self-assessment: occupation knowledge	
Definition of occupation and its defining features	1 2 3 4 5
The specific relationships between occupation, health, and well-being	1 2 3 4 5
Occupation analysis, especially how thorough analyses inform health and well-being outcomes	1 2 3 4 5
The occupation–environment transaction, from macro (geopolitical) to micro (personal) levels	1 2 3 4 5
The ways in which the environment elicits which capacities and abilities are needed for an occupation, e.g., motor, sensory, affective, cognitive, spiritual. Recognizing there is no required set of capacities for a given occupation	1 2 3 4 5

Table 2.1 (Continued)

How context acts as barriers and enablers to occupational engagement, sometimes both simultaneously	1 2 3 4 5
How the transactions between person factors, contexts, and occupations give rise to and suppress occupational performance, engagement, and occupational experience	1 2 3 4 5
Occupational justice	1 2 3 4 5
Occupational experience distinguished from occupational performance and engagement	1 2 3 4 5
The collective or social nature of all occupation	1 2 3 4 5
Meaning as a fluid element of occupation as occupation changes over time or changes in performance	1 2 3 4 5
Models, theories, and research that explicitly support the occupation–health–well-being connection	1 2 3 4 5
Designing learning that helps students create experiences for clients to engage in occupations and explain how the occupations directly support health and well-being	1 2 3 4 5

1 indicates little to no exposure; 5 indicates extensive knowledge or experience

CONCLUSION

Occupation is at the core of occupational therapy and so it is at the core of occupational therapy education. Occupation and its relationship to health and well-being are complex. We need instructional processes that require students to grapple with these complexities so that they can uphold the complexity of the concept at the heart of our contribution to people and society. This work doesn't fall to a single course or content area. Instead, it's a shared responsibility across the curriculum. Regardless of one's area of expertise, every educator plays a role in helping students see how all topics relate to occupation. For some, this might involve revisiting those connections themselves and then creating learning experiences for students to also do so. A deep and ever evolving expertise in occupation is a foundation for reaping the benefits of the SCIL-OT Model.

REFERENCES

Ambrose, S., Bridges, M., DiPietro, M., Lovett, M., & Norman, M. (2010). *How learning works: Seven research-based principles for smart teaching*. Jossey-Bass.

American Occupational Therapy Association. (2020). Occupational therapy practice framework: Domain and process (4th ed.). *American Journal of Occupational Therapy*, *74*(Suppl. 2), 1–87. https://doi.org/10.5014/ajot.2020.74S2001

Backman, C. L., Christiansen, C. H., Hooper, B. R., Pierce, D., & Price, M. P. (2021). Occupational science concepts essential to occupation-based practice: Development of expert consensus. *American Journal of Occupational Therapy*, *75*(6), 7506205120.

Chapparo, C., Ranka, J., & Nott, M. (2017). Occupational Performance Model (Australia): A description of constructs, structure and propositions. In M. Curtin, M. Egan, & J. Adams (Eds.), *Occupational therapy for people experiencing illness, injury or impairment: Promoting occupation and participation* (pp. 134–147). Elsevier.

Molineux, M. (2009). The nature of occupation. In M. Curtin, M. Molineux, & J. Supyk-Mellson (Eds.), *Occupational therapy and physical dysfunction: Enabling occupation* (6th ed., pp. 17–26). Elsevier.

Pierce, D. (2012). Promise. *Journal of Occupational Science*, *19*(4), 298–311. https://doi.org/10.1080/14427591.2012.667778

Polatajko, H., Davis, J., Stewart, D., Cantin, N., Amoroso, B., Purdie, L., & Zimmerman, D. (2007). Specifying the domain of concern: Occupation as core. In E. Townsend & H. Polatajko (Eds.), *Enabling occupation II: Advancing an occupational therapy vision for health, well-being, & justice through occupation* (pp. 13–36). Canadian Association of Occupational Therapists.

Polatajko, H., Davis, J., Stewart, D., Cantin, N., Amoroso, B., Purdie, L., & Zimmerman, D. (2013). Specifying the domain of concern: Occupation as core. In E. Townsend & H. Polatajko (Eds.), *Enabling occupation II: Advancing an occupational therapy vision for health, well-being, & justice through occupation* (2nd ed., pp. 13–36). Canadian Association of Occupational Therapists.

Wilcock, A., & Hocking, C. (2024). *An occupational perspective of health*. Routledge.

Yerxa, E. (1988). Oversimplification: The hobgoblin of theory and practice in occupational therapy. *Canadian Journal of Occupational Therapy*, *55*(1), 5–6.

Chapter 3

The Origins, Evolution, and Education Theories Informing the SCIL-OT Model

INTRODUCTION

Because occupation is the core subject of occupational therapy, it naturally follows that it should also be central to occupational therapy education. As discussed in Chapters 1 and 2, this foundational idea shapes the SCIL-OT Model and its emphasis on helping students make meaningful connections to the concept of occupation. The purpose of this chapter is to trace the origins and evolution of the SCIL-OT Model, including how its key concepts and assumptions were selected, and to introduce three educational theories that support and illuminate its structure: idea-based learning, integrative learning, and transformative learning.

The development of the SCIL-OT Model aligns with the American Occupational Therapy Association's (AOTA, 2018) educational research agenda, which identified theory-building as a priority for advancing occupational therapy education. According to the agenda, theory-building research involves clarifying core concepts in educational practice, exploring how these concepts interact to support student learning, and identifying the learning outcomes most relevant to occupational therapy education. The agenda outlines three goals for theory-building:

(1) To develop profession-specific theories for occupational therapy education and research
(2) To test these theories through research
(3) To rigorously define how educational theories and approaches fit the unique context of the profession (AOTA, 2018, p. 1)

This view of theory-building is also consistent with Lynham's (2013) definition, which describes it as an "ongoing process of producing, confirming, applying, adapting, and refining . . . explanations and understandings of how something works" (pp. 32–33). The development of the SCIL-OT Model roughly followed the

DOI: 10.4324/9781003635628-4

phases Lynham identified: conceptualization, operationalization, confirmation-disconfirmation, and application. These phases are not strictly linear; rather, they are iterative and often occur simultaneously. We refer to these phases throughout the chapter as we describe the model's development.

Throughout this chapter, the use of first-person singular refers to Dr. Barbara Hooper. The use of first-person plural, unless otherwise noted, refers to the authors collectively.

OBJECTIVES

This chapter will help educators to:

1. Explain the theory-building research process from which the SCIL-OT Model evolved.
2. Elucidate three educational theories that inform and support the SCIL-OT Model: idea-based learning, integrative learning, and transformative learning.
3. Clarify how these theories are related and mutually fortifying.
4. Describe views of learning and knowledge that (a) the theories advance and (b) the SCIL-OT Model presupposes.

EVOLUTION AND DEVELOPMENT OF THE SCIL-OT MODEL

We use Lynham's (2013) four phases of theory-building research—conceptualization, operationalization of concepts, application, and refinement—to explain the development of the SCIL-OT model.

Conceptualization

The SCIL-OT Model originated when I was invited to join a Curriculum Mentor initiative of the American Occupational Therapy Foundation (AOTF). At that time, scholars in occupational therapy and occupational science in the United States began using the phrases occupation-centered practice and occupation-centered education (Wood, 1998a, 1998b). These phrases were meant to remind practitioners and educators to focus their efforts with clients and students on the primary aspect of health and well-being that occupational therapy addresses: optimal access to and engagement in occupation. While a few studies were beginning to explore the features of occupation-centered practice, there appeared to be no parallel efforts aimed at clarifying the features of occupation-centered education.

I was so energized by the Curriculum Mentors work that I completely changed my dissertation proposal to conduct an immersive instrumental case study of a program identified at the time as a leader in occupation-centered education. That study involved eight weeks of observing and recording class sessions, reviewing curricular artifacts, and conducting interviews with educators, including video elicitation interviews. Data analysis involved an iterative process of coding and engaging deeply with the education literature to identify explanatory frameworks that could shed light on the practices I was observing, hearing about, and experiencing. Two theoretical frameworks made the data from my dissertation research come alive.

The first theoretical framework was Palmer's (2007, 2017) idea of *subject-centered learning* from the field of education. According to Palmer, subject-centered learning refers to a process in which educators place a 'third thing' (i.e., something other than instructors or students) at the center of teaching and learning. That third thing is the core subject a discipline exists to study, develop, and impact in society. In Palmer's view, when the knowledge of instructors is placed at the center of teaching and learning, content may be portrayed as objective, fixed, and complete. When the experiences of students are placed at the center, content may be portrayed as relativistic and open to any meanings that students ascribe to it—without critical evaluation. The potential for both extremes can be avoided, however, by placing a discipline's core subject at the center of teaching and learning. Ongoing engagement with the core subject mirrors the process of knowledge development, in which what is known about the subject is continually being revealed in and for particular sociocultural contexts. For me, thinking about occupation-centered education as a community gathered around a subject offers a way to both affirm occupation as central to occupational therapy and recognize that its meaning, and enactment must be continually shaped in and for diverse cultural contexts.

Palmer's portrayal of knowledge about core subjects as perpetually being created in and for communities led to the adoption of a second key theoretical framework for the SCIL-OT Model: the theory of self-authorship from constructive developmental psychology, which is part of a larger body of work on transformative learning (Baxter Magolda, 2008, 2020; Kegan, 2018). From a constructive developmental perspective, the complexities of life—and of occupational therapy practice—require that one's beliefs about knowledge, or epistemology, shift from viewing knowledge as static and received from experts to understanding it as dynamic and co-constructed with others in particular contexts. Such a shift is essential because students and instructors are essentially constructing knowledge when they engage in learning processes designed to help students make connections between multiple topics and the core subject of their field. That is, connection-making is knowledge generation, requiring a view of knowledge as always being constructed. Transformative learning, therefore, helped to explain the epistemological foundations of the eventual SCIL-OT Model.

My dissertation research was integral to the conceptualization phase of theory-building. The study's data and theoretical frameworks helped to articulate the model's key assumptions, core concepts and their transactions, and guiding principles (Box 3.1). These early elements were subsequently refined over two decades of operationalization, research, application, and dialogue—to which we (all three authors), as well as other colleagues, education scholars, and graduate students, contributed substantially.

BOX 3.1 CONCEPTUALIZATION PHASE OF THEORY-BUILDING: RESULTS FROM DISSERTATION RESEARCH

Assumptions of the SCIL-OT Model

- Professions have core subjects
- Much of educational content is not profession specific
- The core subject modifies the meaning of topics and how/why they are learned
- Professional and institutional contexts shape what topics are taught and how

Key Concepts of the SCIL-OT Model

- Core Subject
- Topics
- Knowledge Community
- Subject-centered Learning
- Integrative Learning
- Transformative Learning

Key Transactions Among the Concepts

- Specific Occupations-to-Dynamics of Occupation
- Core Subject-to-Topics
- Topics-to-Other Topics

- Knowledge Community Members-to Other Members
- Knowledge Community-to-Core Subject

Principles That Guide Application of the Model

- The core subject of a field is the core subject of teaching and learning
- The core subject is different from the topics that are taught
- Learning a field's core subject takes place in an intentional community
- Instructional design targets learning "on-the-lines"

Ongoing conceptualization of the SCIL-OT Model has involved elaborating the concept of subject-centered learning, as well as the model's elements and theoretical foundations. For example, several fields have a similar concept to subject-centered learning, though they use different terminology. The concept of idea-based learning from education, disciplinary knowledge from nursing, and discipline-based education from the Science, Technology, Engineering, and Math fields all helped deepen how subject-centered learning is portrayed in the SCIL-OT Model. The process of linking topics to the core subject was further clarified through the work of the Carnegie Foundation for the Advancement of Teaching on integrative learning (Huber, Brown, Hutchings, et al., 2007). I came to see that helping students create these linkages within the SCIL-OT Model was highly compatible with integrative learning principles. This compatibility led to the inclusion of integrative learning as another theory that supports the SCIL-OT Model. Integrative learning captured more of the ontological foundations of the model, portraying the nature of reality as a transactional web.

Operationalization

Operationalization involves the creation of propositions that take the form of "if–then" statements, which can be verified through research and scholarship. Through my research, dialogue with educators, and classroom observation, I developed the following tentative propositions:

- If topics are linked to the core subject of occupation, then that connection will be explicit and identifiable in teaching (verbal and written).
- If learning about occupation occurs through engagement in a community, then connections to a knowledge community will be observable.
- If learning about occupation occurs through personal connection, then self-exploration will be present as a learning strategy.

- If topics are taught in direct relation to the core subject of occupation, then the learning of those topics will be observably different than if they are taught in a stand-alone fashion.
- If students learn topics in direct connection to the core subject, then attention to the core subject will be identifiable in their practices and client outcomes.

Guided by one or more of these propositions, subsequent studies variously explored or investigated the following:

- The model's theoretical foundations (Hooper, 2006; Hooper et al., 2014)
- The topography of occupational therapy education in relation to occupation and other features (e.g., Hooper et al., 2014; Roberts et al., 2020)
- The prevalence of the model's elements in teaching stories, video, and artifacts (Brown et al., 2016, 2017; Musick, 2015)
- The utility of the model to educators (Barth, 2026; Hooper & Barth, 2017; Evenson & Hooper, 2019; Hooper & Brown, 2017; Zorn & Hooper, 2017)
- The processes educators use to connect multiple domains of knowledge (Hooper et al., 2014)
- The processes educators use to center teaching and learning on the core subject of occupation (e.g., Krishnagiri et al., 2017; Price et al., 2017)

Box 3.2 offers a partial list of findings from research and application that shaped and continue to shape the model's development. All references to educators in Box 3.2 refer to occupational therapy educators.

BOX 3.2 OPERATIONALIZATION PHASE OF THEORY-BUILDING: KEY CHANGES THROUGH RESEARCH

- In occupational therapy education, the integration of multiple topics was found to be extensive, which supports the principle of "teaching on-the-lines" in the SCIL-OT Model.
- The most frequent connections that educators emphasized were connections of topics to other topics and connections of learners to the knowledge community.
- Fewer connections were made between topics and occupation.
- When educators linked topics to occupation, they frequently described how a topic, such as a health condition, impacted specific occupations such as activities of daily living.

- Educators emphasized fewer connections between specific occupations and health and well-being.
- The knowledge community was the foremost focus in how educators described their teaching. Hence, the quality of connections among students and between students and educators predominantly distinguished satisfying from dissatisfying teaching experiences.
- Educators found that the model's concepts and linkages had high utility for their teaching and instructional design.
- The model served as a reminder to educators to highlight occupation in academic, practice, and client education contexts.
- Practice educators suggested substituting the term "skill" for the term "topics."

Application and Refinement

A powerful shaper of the SCIL-OT Model has been its direct application to educators' teaching practices. Over 400 educators from the United States (predominantly), Canada, South Africa, Japan, Ireland, and Australia participated in summer institutes sponsored by the Center for Occupational Therapy Education. *Together with other experienced educators—including the co-authors of this book—I collaboratively designed and led these workshops*. Their purpose was to help educators actively apply the SCIL-OT Model to their specific academic courses and instructional designs. Attendees, for example, evaluated their courses for how explicitly occupation appeared in objectives, assignments, and assessment tools and designed strategies for strengthening the principles of the SCIL-OT Model in their courses.

The inquiry, dialogue, and application of the model that took place in these institutes are consistent with Neumann's (2009) notion of scholarship as representational knowledge construction. In other words, scholars refine models, theories, and concepts as they create representations of knowledge for others, who in turn engage with those representations through dialogue and learning activities. Such social engagement further refines the knowledge under consideration.

Box 3.3 provides highlights of changes to the model over several iterations of the theory-building phases above.

BOX 3.3 APPLICATION AND REFINEMENT PHASES OF THEORY-BUILDING: EXAMPLES OF KEY CHANGES TO THE SCIL-OT MODEL THROUGH ITS IMPLEMENTATION

- Created several iterations of the model's graphic.
- Added the element and principle related to contexts.
- Broadened exploration of the model's utility to practice educators.
- Redefined the element "topic" to include skills and theories.
- Studied the use of the graphic as a facilitation tool for conversation and mutual goal-setting with students on fieldwork and with clients.
- Created two dimensions to the core subject, specific occupations and dynamics of occupation.
- Expanded the theoretical frameworks underpinning the model.
- Incorporated more interdisciplinary work to explain subject-centered learning.

In the next section, we describe in more detail three theoretical frameworks that help explain the learning foundations of the SCIL-OT Model: idea-based learning, integrative learning, and transformative learning.

THEORETICAL FOUNDATIONS OF THE SCIL-OT MODEL

Idea-based learning explains why it is essential to anchor learning in the big ideas of a professional discipline and supports using a discipline's core subject as a particularly powerful anchor. *Integrative learning* broadly illuminates connection-making as a source of learning. *Transformative learning* refers to acquiring beliefs about knowledge that make connection-making—and therefore learning—possible. As their names imply, each of these theoretical frameworks is fundamentally concerned with learning.

In relation to the SCIL-OT Model, we define learning as the actions and processes through which students develop knowledge, skills, and attitudes that, taken together, enable them to connect specific occupations to the dynamics of occupation, connect salient topics to occupation, connect topics to other topics, connect their own experiences to occupation, and so forth. Furthermore, learning involves actions and processes through which students justify how the connections they have drawn support their selected courses of action. Together, these three theoretical frameworks conceptually support this complex web of connection-making as a foundation for learning in occupational therapy. Each theory is introduced in the sections that follow.

Idea-Based Learning

Because students are often overwhelmed by all they must learn, idea-based learning is based on the presumption that learning is facilitated when students link individual topics or bits of content to a central organizing idea—or to a few big ideas—that characterize a field (Hansen, 2012; Wiggins & McTighe, 2005). Proponents of idea-based learning accordingly draw important distinctions between the basic ideas taught in a field and the field's big ideas (Hansen, 2011; Wiggins & McTighe, 2005). Basic ideas refer to a body of facts, definitions, skills, and accurate performances or competencies. Among many possibilities, examples of basic ideas that occupational therapy students might learn include developmental milestones of young children, research methods, musculoskeletal structure and function, and sensory integration. In contrast to these basic ideas, big ideas are those that have endured in a field—even as they continue to be discovered, elaborated, and renewed through inquiry.

Table 3.1 illustrates three ways scholars in occupational therapy have conceptualized the big ideas of the field: as the profession's distinctive ethos, philosophy, and threshold concepts. While named differently, each version points to similar enduring ideas. Because big ideas such as these characterize occupational therapy, they serve as a kind of conceptual Velcro—helping students connect a wide range of topics, transfer learning to practice, and understand what constitutes learning priorities.

Distinguishing basic ideas from big ideas is vital. According to Hansen (2011), a curriculum that clearly draws these distinctions can equip learners to flexibly transfer the core ideas of occupational therapy into varying practice situations. Conversely, a curriculum that does not make these distinctions can leave students overwhelmed by a wide array of discrete facts, skills, and experiences. Moreover, when students do not learn to distinguish basic from big ideas, they may acquire bits of information and discrete competencies yet still lack a cohesive structure for generating deep meaning and contextual understanding. The unfortunate result is that students may neither fully comprehend the distinct value of their professional expertise related to occupation nor develop a correspondingly strong and clear professional identity.

Table 3.1 Three examples of how scholars have compiled the big ideas of occupational therapy.

Compilations of the big ideas of occupational therapy	**Big ideas**
Ethos of Occupational Therapy (Peloquin, 2005)	• Time, place, and circumstance open paths to occupation • Occupation fosters dignity, competence, and health • Occupational therapy is a personal engagement • Caring and helping are vital to the work • Effective practice is artistry and science
Philosophy of Occupational Therapy (Hooper & Wood, 2023)	• Ever-changing humans, interconnected with ever-changing environments, occupy time with ever-changing occupations, and thereby transform—and are transformed by—their actions, environments, and states of health. • Knowledge about occupation is primary and serves as the key subject that integrates all other knowledge and clarifies the desired consequences of action. • Practice involves collaboration with clients-and-environments-as-a-whole to achieve meaningful and satisfying participation in occupation and thereby optimal potential, well-being, and health.
Threshold Concepts (Rodger & Turpin, 2011; Fortune & Kennedy-Jones, 2014)	• Purposeful and meaningful occupation • Client-centered practice • Integral nature of theory and practice • Identity as an occupational therapist • Thinking critically • Reasoning and reflection • Occupation and its relationship with health

As former students and now educators, many of us have experienced curricula that do not distinguish the multitude of basic ideas students must learn from the big ideas of occupational therapy. For example, we may have experienced occupational therapy education as traditionally organized into lifespan categories or into the sub-specialties of the field. We may have taken or taught courses focused on pediatrics, adults, or older adults. We may have encountered courses on biomechanics and neuroscience, orthopedic or neurological conditions, or specific person factors like cognition, vision, and sensory processing. We may also have taken or taught courses organized by broad skill areas such as assessment, intervention, or environmental adaptations, or by more specific skill areas such as orthotics or physical agent modalities. When used as anchors for curriculum and course design, these content areas can appear to students as if they constitute the big ideas of occupational therapy—that is, the profession's essential logic. Yet these content areas actually comprise basic ideas, and the emphasis placed on them may keep the big ideas of the profession hidden from students.

Many of us have grown so accustomed to curricula and courses being organized around basic ideas that it can be difficult to imagine a compelling alternative—one that could, in fact, enhance learning. Yet such an alternative does exist. Consistent with idea-based learning, that alternative is to organize curricula and courses around the big ideas of occupational therapy and to use these big ideas as powerful pedagogical tools. For example, some courses may be developed around the idea that people experience health and well-being in direct relation to their access to and participation in occupation. Other courses might be developed around the idea that loss of occupation is a determinant of diminished health and well-being, followed by courses centered on the big idea that occupational therapy exists to ensure the just distribution of occupational engagement in society.

If this alternative approach is employed, students can still develop important proficiencies in performing discrete skills, working with people of all ages and abilities, and practicing in various sub-specialty areas. In other words, they can still acquire the competencies often associated with more traditional curriculum design. In addition, organizing curricula and courses around the big ideas of occupational therapy can help students connect the particular proficiencies they have acquired with increasingly precise and informed conceptual understandings of the profession. This kind of connection-making can deepen student learning and enhance their ability to apply what they've learned across diverse practice contexts.

Seminal works in the education literature support the idea that using big ideas as pedagogical tools facilitates important learning outcomes (e.g., Bain, 2004; Bransford et al., 2016; Bruner, 2009; Donovan & Bransford, 2005; Paul & Elder, 2013). For instance, according to Bransford et al. (2016), authors of *How People Learn*, competence as a learning outcome depends on students being able to understand topics within the context of a larger conceptual framework—namely, the core subject and big ideas of the field. When students learn individual topics in a way that is detached from such a framework, they may succeed on exams yet remain poorly equipped to apply the logic of their field in multiple practice contexts.

The SCIL-OT Model can remind educators to help students connect a multitude of basic ideas to deep understandings of the big ideas of occupational therapy—especially its core subject of occupation. Because accreditation standards require it, all occupational therapy education programs, of course, teach students *about* occupation. Yet if students are taught only *about* occupation, it can become just another basic idea. Idea-based learning helps us, as educators, distinguish between teaching about occupation and positioning occupation as the idea at the center of all learning.

Integrative Learning

Whereas idea-based learning specifically focuses on using the big ideas of a field to facilitate learning, integrative learning broadly illuminates the educational value of connection-making. In the health professions, integrative learning refers to teaching and learning processes that educators intentionally design to foster connections among diverse phenomena. Hooper et al. (2014, p. 470) proposed that these phenomena include the

> *core subject, perspective and habits of mind of the profession, abstract knowledge, responsible application of concrete skills, the subjective experiences and objective needs of service recipients, germane evidence, professional reasoning, relevant features of the practice situation, and the experience level and identity of the practitioner.*

Connection-making among such diverse phenomena supports learning because it reflects

1) the interconnected nature of all phenomena.
2) the mindset and skills that professionals need to address complex problems.
3) how occupational therapy practitioners think in practice.

With respect to the interconnected nature of all phenomena, Palmer et al. (2010) suggested that most, if not all, phenomena that students learn are by nature relational or ecological. Phenomena exist in webs of relation to other phenomena. Students learn when they connect the phenomena that comprise such webs because this connection-making mirrors how things ultimately exist and function—namely, as dynamic, integrated wholes.

From a learning perspective, dynamic, integrated wholes encompass both external and internal phenomena. Palmer et al. (2010) argued that inner phenomena are vital to learning—especially the personal elements of students' own beliefs, values, and longings. Learning occurs when students form these elements into coherent meaning systems that align with their outer experiences and explorations. In short, learning occurs when students connect who they are with what they do. Moreover, to integrate who they are with what they do in a meaningful way, students must develop capacities for critical self-reflection. These capacities include the ability both to step back and critically examine one's beliefs and to revise those beliefs as new circumstances, experiences, knowledge, and understandings emerge. According to Palmer et al. (2010), exercising these capacities facilitates learning because it occurs where "meaning and purpose are tightly woven with intellect and action" and "compassion and care are infused with insight and knowledge" (p. 56).

With respect to the mindset and skills needed to address complex problems, higher education scholars promote integrative learning because societal problems are too complex to be solved by a few individuals considering only a narrow range of topics (Palmer et al., 2010; Huber et al., 2013). Rather, solutions to complex societal problems emerge as many different people and disciplines continuously experiment with connecting diverse areas of knowledge. Connection-making is thus vital for learning because it reflects the mindset and skills that citizens and professionals in contemporary societies need. It follows that if students are to learn how to address societal problems, then higher education must engage them in collaborative experiences of complex connection-making.

A parallel argument can be made for integrative learning in occupational therapy specifically. Occupational therapy students must learn how to address highly complex problems related to people's occupations and lives. The complexity of these problems cannot be adequately addressed by students who consider only what they already know about a few disconnected topics. Rather, solutions require that students collaboratively experiment with interconnecting their existing knowledge across diverse topics while also exploring new knowledge. Therefore, educators must engage students in experiences that require dynamic connection-making as a source of learning.

We believe that connection-making is a powerful source of learning for occupational therapy students precisely because it reflects how occupational therapists understand the profession and its core subject of occupation. To our knowledge, no well-established or widely accepted non-ecological theories, models, or perspectives currently hold significant influence in the profession. Rather, what is pervasive are ecological theories, models, and perspectives on occupation and the occupational therapy process (see, for instance, Cutchin & Dickie, 2012; Hasselkus & Dickie, 2021; Iwama, 2006).

Thus, connection-making is also a powerful source of learning because it reflects how occupational therapy practitioners think in practice. Consider, for instance, Mattingly and Fleming's (1994) groundbreaking study of clinical reasoning in occupational therapy. These scholars found that expert practitioners quite automatically and quickly pieced together a great deal of information relevant to complex clinical situations. Their well-developed habits of connection-making helped them customize clinical approaches for different clients with different life circumstances. As described by Schell and Schell (2017), the clinical reasoning of occupational therapists involves ongoing connection-making among diverse theoretical, scientific, narrative, pragmatic, and ethical elements of a given practice situation. Because each practice situation is unique—regardless of how seemingly routine—connection-making comprises one of the profession's most fundamental and essential reasoning skills (Hooper & Wood, 2023). Therefore, students learn to think like practitioners when they engage in collaborative processes of connection-making across diverse areas of knowledge.

It is little wonder, then, that we as educators often say we want students to 'put the pieces together' or 'connect the dots.' By putting pieces together or connecting dots, we essentially mean that we want students to begin thinking like highly effective practitioners. Such practitioners continuously make a myriad of connections—linking their knowledge of guiding theory and evidence; the occupational issues, goals, personal contexts, and environments of their clients; the constraints and opportunities of their practice settings; and many other factors. We therefore want students to demonstrate the profession's most fundamental reasoning skill: linking numerous factors to enable occupation. We also want students to critically reflect on the congruence between their own values and belief systems and those of the profession. Such critical self-reflection is essential if students are to connect their personal and emerging professional identities with their particular actions as developing members of the occupational therapy profession.

Transformative Learning

Transformative learning refers to the processes by which students' assumptions about knowledge—and about themselves in relation to knowledge and others—transform in ways that make connection-making, and therefore learning, possible (Baxter Magolda & King, 2012). Baxter Magolda (2023) used narrative research to identify a developmental progression of beliefs about knowledge that many students and young adults undergo. She referred to these stages of belief as "ways of knowing." Students may enter higher education or graduate school with the belief that knowledge is certain and fixed, existing somewhere external to themselves. From this perspective, students expect instructors to deliver knowledge as clearly as possible so they can receive it efficiently and demonstrate it competently. At this stage, students do not typically value learning from others in self-directed, problem-based groups. Baxter Magolda refers to this stage of belief—or way of knowing—as "absolute knowing."

However, the work of integrative learning is challenging, if not impossible, for students who rely on absolute knowing. It is impossible because, from an absolute knowing lens, there is no need to build connections or construct meaning. From this perspective, knowledge is presumed to be fixed and external—'out there,' so to speak. As a result, students who rely on absolute knowing believe they must receive knowledge from others rather than participate in its construction.

Therefore, another way of knowing is required if students are to engage in integrative and idea-based learning. They need a way of knowing that embraces knowledge as uncertain, evolving, and constructed through the active integration of diverse topics and contexts. They also need to see themselves as knowledge creators—individuals who participate in constructing knowledge collaboratively with others. Baxter Magolda (2023) refers to this set of beliefs as "contextual knowing": the ability to critically evaluate a situation, assemble knowledge in and for that situation, and explain and justify why a particular approach is more appropriate than others to meet the needs of that context.

In moving from absolute knowing to contextual knowing, students often progress through two interim stages known as transitional knowing and independent knowing (Baxter Magolda & King, 2004). In transitional knowing, students' beliefs about knowledge begin to shift—they allow for some uncertainty, while still believing that most knowledge is certain and held by experts. In independent knowing, students' beliefs swing toward relativism. As they begin to see more knowledge as uncertain, they may conclude that if knowledge is not fixed or held exclusively by experts, then any opinion is equally valid. Educators create learning contexts that challenge students to move beyond this stage toward contextual knowing. Achieving contextual knowing is essential because the complexities of life—and of occupational therapy practice—demand the ability to examine situations from multiple viewpoints, consider desired outcomes and influential factors, and integrate those considerations with students' experiences, ethics, intuitions, and sociocultural contexts to take skillful action.

The process of gradually moving from absolute knowing to contextual knowing is referred to as transformative learning (Baxter Magolda & King, 2012). When students begin to perceive knowledge as contextual, they understand it as naturally tentative and fluid—constructed through experience, sound judgment, evidence, and situational factors. At the same time, students shift from seeing themselves as recipients of knowledge to viewing themselves as active co-creators and evaluators of knowledge within the inquiry practices of a professional community.

We easily recognize these stages of epistemological development in our experiences as occupational therapy educators. Many students enter occupational therapy programs with absolute assumptions about knowledge. For instance, students often assume that the profession of occupational therapy is a 'finished' product—something 'out there'—and that instructors can simply take the knowledge they need off a metaphorical shelf and hand it down intact. To learn, they expect instructors to present that knowledge in a clear, simple, and organized form so they can receive it, mirror it back as given, and thus 'have it.'

When students discover that knowledge in and about occupational therapy is in process and continuously being developed, they can be quite surprised—even frustrated. Students' personal learning histories may have conditioned them to focus on basic ideas, facts, principles, definitions, skills, and competencies—without needing to actively construct, in collaboration with others, the connections between basic ideas and the field's big ideas. In other words, students may arrive in our programs believing that knowledge is fixed, educators convey it, and they receive it. This belief system is, in essence, their way of knowing—what Baxter Magolda (2020) refers to as "absolute knowing." When we as educators create opportunities for students to actively assemble knowledge into multiple possible solutions—not just one—to various conceptual and tactical problems, students' beliefs begin to shift. This shift is often tacit; students may surprise themselves by having completed and presented a case study, a research project, a new program, or a unique intervention plan. These types of learning activities can embed the tenets of contextual knowing and, in doing so, promote transformation.

Therefore, transformative learning offers a third theoretical framework that supports the SCIL-OT Model and underpins both idea-based and integrative learnings. To fully engage in integrative learning—connecting topics to the big ideas of occupation—students must embrace knowledge as a puzzle they are constantly assembling and reassembling. We, as educators, design learning experiences that require students to connect multiple elements. In doing so, we create contexts that encourage students to view knowledge as fluid and situational—a perspective necessary for addressing the complexities of practice.

Altogether, given their shared emphasis on connection-making, the three theoretical frameworks identified in this chapter are closely related and mutually reinforcing. Whereas idea-based learning helps explain why it is crucial to anchor learning around a field's big concepts, integrative learning underscores the broader value of connection-making as a powerful learning tool. Transformative learning, in turn, identifies the range of students' possible beliefs about the nature of knowledge and how they might grow—from viewing knowledge as absolute and handed down by experts to seeing it as dynamic and contextually situated. Together, these theories illuminate how we can help students develop habits of deep and persistent connection-making related to occupational therapy's core subject of occupation, its big ideas, and their wise application in practice.

CONCLUSION

The SCIL-OT Model has been developed and refined through systematic processes of conceptualization, operationalization, application, and refinement. As noted in the preface, the model remains a work in progress. We hope this book invites and inspires education scholars to apply the model, study it across diverse contexts, and continue improving it as a tool for designing occupation-centered curricula and instruction.

Chapter 4 introduces the model itself. The SCIL-OT Model adopts an ecological view of occupational therapy and its core subject, occupation. It is grounded in the belief that occupational therapy involves a complex web of interconnected phenomena—phenomena that students come to understand through learning experiences that intentionally prompt them to continually discover and draw meaningful interconnections.

Ideally, throughout their education, students come to see progressively clearer and more meaningful connections between occupation and their personal development, health, well-being, and sense of meaning. They also begin to connect seemingly disparate topics in ways that deepen their understanding of occupation. And, we hope, they come to recognize connections among diverse communities—unified in their efforts to illuminate aspects of occupation in socially relevant contexts.

REFERENCES

American Occupational Therapy Association. (2018). Occupational therapy education research agenda–revised. *American Journal of Occupational Therapy*, *72*(Suppl. 2), 7212420070p1–7212420070p5. https://doi.org/10.5014/ajot.2018.72S218

Bain, K. (2004). *What the best college teachers do*. Harvard University Press.

Barth, D. C. (2016). *Exploring the applicability and utility of a subject centered integrative learning model in fieldwork education* (Order No. 10156640). ProQuest Dissertations & Theses Global (1837384201).

Baxter Magolda, M. B., & King, P. M. (Eds.). (2004). *Learning partnerships: Theory and models of practice to educate for self-authorship*. Stylus.

Baxter Magolda, M. B. (2008). Three elements of self-authorship. *Journal of college student development, 49*(4), 269–284.

Baxter Magolda, M. B. & King, P. M. (2012). *Assessing Meaning Making and Self-Authorship: Theory, Research, and Application*: ASHE Higher Education Report 38: 3. John Wiley & Sons.

Baxter Magolda, M. B. (2023). *Making their own way: Narratives for transforming higher education to promote self-development*. Routledge.

Bransford, J., Brown, A., & Cocking, R. (2016). *How people learn: Brain, mind, experience and school*. National Academy Press.

Brown, A., Hooper, B., Barth, D., & Zorn, A. (2017). Operationalizing occupation-centered education: Exploring the subject-centered integrative learning model in academic education. *American Journal of Occupational Therapy*, *71*(4_Suppl. 1), 7111505158p7111505151. https://doi.org/10.5014/ajot.2017.71S1-PO7145

Bruner, J. S. (2009). *The process of education*. Harvard University Press.

Cutchin, M. P., & Dickie, V. A. (2012). *Transactional perspectives on occupation*. Springer.

Donovan, S., & Bransford, J. (2005). *How students learn*. National Academies Press.

Evenson, M., & Hooper, B. (2019). *Exploring the applicability and utility of a subject centered integrative learning model among fieldwork educators and students* [Unpublished manuscript]. MGH Institute of Health Professions.

Fortune, T., & Kennedy-Jones, M. (2014). Occupation and its relationship with health and well-being: The threshold concept for occupational therapy. *Australian Occupational Therapy Journal*, *61*(5), 293–298.

Hansen, E. J. (2011). *Idea-based learning: A course design process to promote conceptual understanding*. Stylus Publishing.

Hasselkus, B. R., & Dickie, V. (2021). *The meaning of everyday occupation* (2nd ed.). Slack Incorporated.

Hooper, B. R. (2006). Beyond active learning: A case study of teaching practices in an occupation-centered curriculum. *American Journal of Occupational Therapy*, *60*, 551–562.

Hooper, B. R., & Barth, D. (2017, October). Exploring the applicability and utility of the subject-centered integrative learning model in academic education. Paper presented at the American Occupational Therapy Association Education Summit, Philadelphia, PA.

Hooper, B. R., & Brown, A. (2017, October). Exploring the applicability and utility of the subject-centered integrative learning model in academic education. Paper presented at the American Occupational Therapy Association Education Summit, Philadelphia, PA.

Hooper, B. R., Greene, D., & Sample, P. L. (2014). Exploring features of integrative teaching through a microanalysis of connection-making processes in a health sciences curriculum. *Advances in Health Sciences Education*, *19*(4), 451–470. https://doi.org/10.1007/s10459-013-9481-5

Hooper, B., & Wood, W. (2023). A philosophy of occupational therapy: A framework for practice. In G. Gillen & C. Brown (Eds.), *Willard & Spackman's occupational therapy* (14th ed., pp. 38–53). Wolters Kluwer/LWW.

Huber, M. T., Brown, C., Hutchings, P., Gale, R., Miller, R., & Breen, M. (2007). *Integrative learning: Opportunities to connect*. Association of American Colleges & Universities and Carnegie Foundation for the Advancement of Teaching.

Huber, M. T., Hutchings, P., Brooker, R., Couch, B., Fisher, M. A., Gale, R. M., Higgs, B., Kremer, G. G., Liu, X., & Maiolatesi, K. (2013). *Connected science: Strategies for integrative learning in college*. Indiana University Press.

Iwama, M. K. (2006). *The Kawa model: Culturally relevant occupational therapy*. Churchill Livingstone Elsevier.

Kegan, R. (2018). What "form" transforms?: A constructive-developmental approach to transformative learning. In K. Illeris (Ed.) *Contemporary theories of learning* (pp. 29–45). Routledge.

Krishnagiri, S., Hooper, B., Price, P., Taff, S. D., & Bilics, A. (2017). Explicit or hidden? Exploring how occupation is taught in occupational therapy curricula in the United States. *American Journal of Occupational Therapy*, *71*(2), 7102230020p7102230021–7102230020p7102230029.

Lynham, S. A. (2013). General method of theory building in applied disciplines. In R. Swanson & T. Chermack (Eds.), *Theory building in applied disciplines*. Berrett-Koehler Publishers.

Mattingly, C., & Fleming, M. H. (1994). *Clinical reasoning: Forms of inquiry in a therapeutic practice*. F. A. Davis.

Musick, L. M. (2015). *Elements of a subject-centered education model in occupational therapy education* (Publication No. Dissertation/Thesis) [Doctoral dissertation, ProQuest Dissertations Publishing]. https://go.exlibris.link/jzfzdRXb

Neumann, A. (2009). *Professing to learn: Creating tenured lives and careers in the American research university*. JHU Press.

Palmer, P. J. (2007). *The courage to teach: Exploring the inner landscape of a teacher's life*. John Wiley & Sons.

Palmer, P. J. (2017). *The courage to teach: Exploring the inner landscape of a teacher's life* (Anniversary ed.). John Wiley & Sons.

Palmer, P. J., Zajonc, A., & Scribner, M. (2010). *The heart of higher education: A call to renewal*. John Wiley & Sons.

Paul, R., & Elder, L. (2013). *Critical thinking: Tools for taking charge of your professional and personal life*. Pearson Education.

Peloquin, S. M. (2005). Embracing our ethos, reclaiming our heart. *American Journal of Occupational Therapy*, *59*(6), 611–625.

Price, P., Hooper, B., Krishnagiri, S., Taff, S. D., & Bilics, A. (2017). A way of seeing: How occupation is portrayed to students when taught as a concept beyond its use in therapy. *American Journal of Occupational Therapy*, *71*(4), 7104230010p7104230011–7104230010p7104230019.

Roberts, M., Hooper, B., & Molineux, M. (2020). Occupational therapy entry-level education scholarship in Australia from 2000 to 2019: A systematic mapping review. *Australian Occupational Therapy Journal*, *67*(4), 373–395.

Rodger, S., & Turpin, M. (2011). Using threshold concepts to transform entry level curricula. *Research and Development in Higher Education*, *34*, 263–274.

Schell, B. A. B., & Schell, J. (2017). *Clinical and professional reasoning in occupational therapy* (2nd ed.). Lippincott Williams & Wilkins.

Wiggins, G. P., & McTighe, J. (2005). *Understanding by design* (2nd ed.). Association for Supervision and Curriculum Development

Wood, W. (1998a). Occupation-centered practice [Special issue]. *American Journal of Occupational Therapy*, *52*(6).

Wood, W. (1998b). Occupation-centered education [Special issue]. *American Journal of Occupational Therapy*, *52*(6).

Zorn, A., & Hooper, B. (2017, October). Exploring the applicability and utility of the subject-centered integrative learning model in client education. Paper presented at the American Occupational Therapy Association Education Summit, Philadelphia, PA.

Chapter 4

The Subject-Centered Integrative Learning Model for Occupational Therapy Education

INTRODUCTION

In Chapter 1, we proposed that occupational therapy exists to oversee and distribute the public good of health and well-being through occupation. We also proposed that best educational practices in occupational therapy are discipline-based, meaning strongly centered on our profession's core subject of occupation and its distinct societal contributions.

In Chapter 2, we explored occupation-centered education more deeply, initiating a discussion that foregrounds not only specific occupations but also the dynamics of occupation.

In Chapter 3, we presented the development of the model and three theoretical perspectives—idea-based learning, transformative learning, and integrative learning—that most centrally inform the SCIL-OT Model.

With this foundation in place, the purpose of Chapter 4 is to present the SCIL-OT Model in full. We provide a brief overview of all five elements of the model and devote the remainder of the chapter to developing each element in depth.

We close each description with the principle that guides the element and identify educational challenges that often arise in relation to it. We also present strategies suggested by the SCIL-OT Model that we and other educators have used to address these teaching and learning challenges.

As you read, consider how each element and its guiding principle show up in your own teaching practice, and how the SCIL-OT Model might support you in addressing persistent challenges.

DOI: 10.4324/9781003635628-5

OBJECTIVES

This chapter will help educators to:

1. Elucidate the elements and principles of occupation-centered education that inform the SCIL-OT Model.
2. Identify commonplace challenges related to educational approaches and teaching methods, for each element of the model.
3. Identify useful strategies for addressing identified challenges, for each element of the model.

INTRODUCING THE SCIL-OT MODEL

As illustrated in Figure 4.1, the SCIL-OT Model comprises five elements. Refer to Figure 4.1 as you read to visualize how these elements interact and support occupation-centered learning.

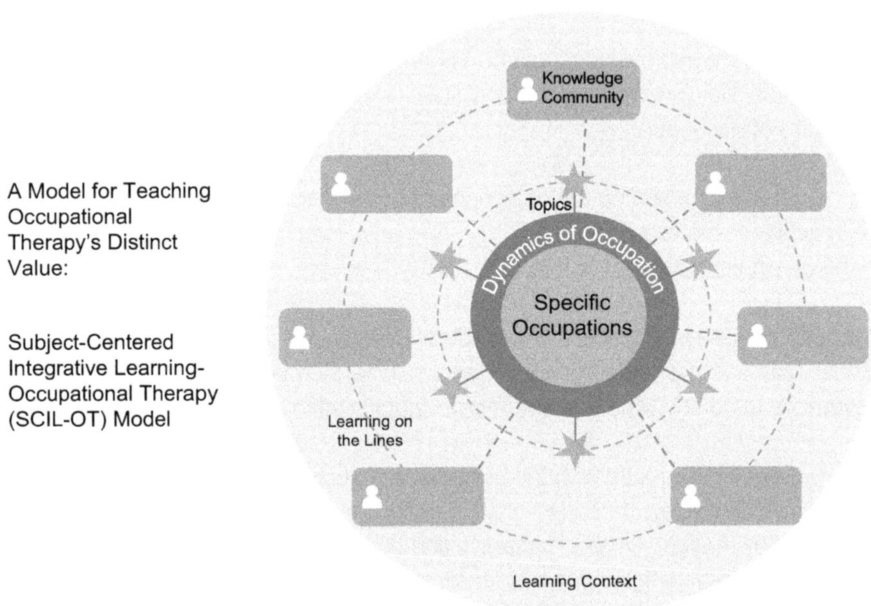

Figure 4.1 Five elements of the Subject-Centered Integrated Learning-Occupational Therapy Model (SCIL-OT): (1) occupation (center circles); (2) topics (stars); (3) the knowledge community (human icons); (4) the learning context (background circle); and (5) the connecting lines (solid and dashed lines).

OVERVIEW OF FIVE ELEMENTS THAT COMPRISE THE SCIL-OT MODEL

Because the model is designed to enhance occupation-centered education, *occupation* comprises its first and most centrally depicted element. A sharp educational focus is placed on two aspects of occupation: specific occupations and the dynamics of occupation.

Specific occupations refer to people's distinct and concrete doings—tasks, activities, and other undertakings that make up daily life. These are commonly categorized broadly within various taxonomies of occupation, such as basic and instrumental activities of daily living, work, education, and play and leisure, among others. They are categorized more specifically when people describe what they want, need, and are expected to do each day or over time; for example, reading, getting and taking groceries to an elderly relative, walking the dog.

The dynamics of occupation refer to the complex transactions from which occupations emerge and the inner workings of specific occupations that impact people's health and well-being.

Topics comprise the second element of the SCIL-OT Model. Topics are broadly defined to include explicit practice-related skills, concepts, facts, theories, attitudes, and dispositions that educators and students collaboratively construct and apply. Topics also encompass areas of emphasis within particular programs, often expressed as curriculum threads, domains, or themes. Examples of such emphases include client-centered practice, ethical practice, evidence-based practice, occupational justice, clinical reasoning, and belonging.

The knowledge community comprises the third element of the SCIL-OT Model. Broadly defined, the knowledge community includes anyone—within or outside the profession—who can help illuminate the core subject of occupation and relevant topics.

Students and educators are vital members, but far from the only ones. Knowledge communities also include authors of books, research studies, theories, and other published works or social media that students engage with. They also include occupational therapists, interdisciplinary colleagues, clients, and others in the client's constellation whom students encounter throughout their education.

The learning context comprises the fourth element of the SCIL-OT Model. It refers to both external and internal influences on curriculum design and implementation.

Context refers to mutually influential factors such as institutional type, size, and priorities, geographical location, program faculty expertise, institution and community partners, marketplace dynamics, financial and learning resources, among others.

In the model, these and other contextual factors work in tandem to shape a distinctive curriculum:

- How occupation is understood
- Which occupations are deemed most relevant
- Which topics are prioritized
- Who is considered part of the knowledge community
- Which teaching approaches and methods are most valued

The connecting lines comprise the fifth element of the SCIL-OT Model. These lines represent where to aim educational approaches and teaching methods. That is, all curriculum design activity across all four levels of curriculum (see Chapter 1) aims to facilitate meaningful connections.

As illustrated in Figure 4.1, types of connection-making include the following:

- Connecting specific occupations and the dynamics of occupation (center circles)
- Connecting topics to occupation (lines from stars to center circles)
- Connecting topics to other topics (lines between stars)
- Connecting personal experience to occupation (lines from rectangles to center circles)
- Connecting members of the knowledge community to what one is learning (lines from rectangles)

The sum of these connections constitutes occupation-centered learning.

The connecting lines are especially critical because the model is based on the presumption that designing a curriculum's educational approaches and teaching methods for connection-making—or *teaching on-the-lines*—is what brings occupation-centered learning alive. Because of these connecting lines, none of the other four elements—occupation, topics, learning context, or knowledge community—are conceived of as separate or stand-alone entities. Instead, the SCIL-OT Model is designed to support educational approaches and teaching methods that are not only explicitly occupation-centered but also highly integrative in nature.

As you reflect on your own teaching, consider: Where are the lines of connection strongest—and where might they be strengthened to bring learning more fully to life?

THE FIVE ELEMENTS OF THE SCIL-OT MODEL IN DEPTH

First Element: Occupation

As the subject at the center—or core—of all occupational therapy education, occupation, comprises the first element of the SCIL-OT Model. The model highlights two dimensions of occupation that educators must consider when designing and implementing curricula—across programs, courses, classroom experiences, and practice education. These dimensions are as follows: (1) specific occupations and (2) the dynamics of occupation (see Figure 4.1).

Specific Occupations

Specific occupations refer to everyday experiences such as dressing, meal preparation, cleaning, caring for others, work, education, shopping, and community mobility. Occupational therapy educators often teach specific occupations in ways that align with the SCIL-OT Model. For example, students may be asked to observe, analyze, adapt, teach their peers, and learn specific occupations.

Educators also guide students to connect specific occupations to client and environment factors, such as how movement, vision, cognition, the physical, social, or virtual contexts impact occupation. Students often use learning resources such as the Occupational Therapy Practice Framework (AOTA, 2020), Enabling Occupation II (Townsend & Polatajko, 2013), and Powerful Practice (Fisher & Marterella, 2019) to support these connections.

In addition, students often learn to consider specific occupations as both an end and a means.

> *As an end, students analyze how impairments (e.g., visual scanning, swallowing, or upper extremity motor control) affect a person's ability to eat, for example, and how to adapt eating to minimize those impacts. They may also learn to teach caregivers strategies that enable clients to eat despite persistent impairments.*

As a means, students explore how the demands of eating can be configured to promote active participation and remediate impairments.

Including specific occupations as one dimension of the core subject reinforces long-standing instructional strategies. However, these strategies alone will not help students fully grasp the complexities of occupation.

The Dynamics of Occupation

The model further guides us to design instruction that helps students develop deep understandings of the relationship between specific occupations and human health and well-being—in other words, the dynamics of occupation. These dynamics help students explain why occupation is a critical factor in health.

Just as in teaching specific occupations, educators commonly draw students' attention to the dynamics of occupation in meaningful ways. For example, many programs include mission and vision statements that emphasize promoting health and well-being through occupation.

We introduce foundational concepts related to the dynamics of occupation such as the following:

- Humans possess an innate, biological need for occupation.
- "Engaging in occupation supports survival, growth, development, health, and well-being" (Hooper & Wood, 2018, p. 46).

We also teach histories, philosophies, research, and theories that expose students to classic and contemporary understandings of occupation and its relationship to health.

Students often engage in reflective learning experiences—such as examining their own occupations and how these have contributed to their capacity development and social connections over time. For example,

- Educators may ask students to write about a time when they experienced occupational disruption and how it affected their physical, mental, and social health, or
- Educators may design assignments that prompt students to evaluate their own health and well-being and create a personal intervention to optimize engagement in occupation during graduate school.

However, students may not always understand the deeper purpose behind these activities. Without clear connections from the learning activity back to the dynamics of occupation, students may struggle to grasp why occupational therapists focus on particular occupations—like eating—in the first place. This limited understanding can make it easier for them to drift away from practices that directly address occupational engagement.

This is why the SCIL-OT Model emphasizes the critical linkages between specific occupations and the dynamics of occupation.

> As you reflect on your curriculum, ask yourself:
>
> - Are students learning how specific occupations relate to health—not just how they're performed?
> - Can students explain the dynamics that make occupation a vital instrument in health, in both positive and negative directions?

Teaching and Learning Focused on the Dynamics Activated by Specific Occupations

The SCIL-OT Model draws our attention to teaching and learning that helps students focus on three key ideas:

- A single occupation is one link in a long chain of related occupations.
- Macro-level contexts influence whether an occupation exists and if it benefits or harms health.
- Specific occupations form the foundation of health and well-being.

A single occupation is one link in a long chain of related occupations. Let's revisit the occupation of eating. It is easy to teach eating as a single occupation. Using the SCIL-OT model, we design learning activities that place eating within a broader chain of food-related occupations—such as growing, harvesting, packaging, transporting, acquiring, preparing, and sharing food. Through intentional learning activities, students discover that supports and challenges across this entire chain may impact the act of eating just as motor capacities like chewing and swallowing do.

We can also design learning activities that explore how eating is typically coordinated with other occupations occurring simultaneously, such as helping others eat, catching up on the news, or connecting with loved ones.

Macro-level contexts influence whether an occupation exists and if it benefits or harms health. By macro contexts, we mean the web of influences that

- give rise to specific occupations in time and place.
- make the doing of occupations possible.
- shape how occupations are performed and experienced.

Examples of these macro-level contexts include the geopolitical, sociocultural, physical, temporal, historical, and technological contexts, among others. Guided by the SCIL-OT Model, we design instruction that helps students explore these macro-level contexts in depth. One helpful tool is the Transactional Model of Occupation (Fisher & Marterella, 2019), which outlines the various elements that influence whether an occupation is available, to whom, how it is performed, and how it is experienced.

Returning to the example of eating, students might examine how each act of eating reflects a unique convergence of these broader occupations and contexts.

To illustrate, occupational scientists Bagatell and Womack (2016) described a course in which students explored the dynamics behind specific occupations, including eating. Students examined sociocultural and geopolitical factors influencing what and how one eats, as well as the social dynamics involved in eating.

After establishing macro influences, students then examined body functions and structures that support eating—such as the digestive, gustatory, olfactory, oral motor, musculoskeletal, and neurologic systems.

Students also explored how these systems themselves vary depending on the eating situation.

Altogether, the SCIL-OT Model's central focus on occupation aligns with many existing and useful educational approaches. At the same time, the model urges us to assess whether—and to what degree—our teaching explicitly links specific occupations with the broader dynamics of occupation.

CONSIDER YOUR OWN TEACHING:

- How do you help students see the layers of context from which everyday occupations like eating arise?

Specific occupations form the foundation of health and well-being. Understanding the dynamic and emergent nature of occupation and how occupations are chained together helps students appreciate the complexity of what people and communities do. However, appreciating complexity is not the same as understanding how and why occupation impacts health. To make that connection clear, educators must integrate knowledge of specific occupations with models of health that reflect an occupational perspective.

One example from our own teaching illustrates this integration. Drawing from Wilcock and Hocking, we use the framework of Doing, Being, Becoming, and Belonging (DB3) to help students explore the health dynamics of occupation.

Students examine how specific occupations contain the elements of DB3. They next correlate the DB3 elements to physical, mental, and social health.

Specifically,

- Doing and Becoming together support physical health and well-being.
- Being and Becoming together promote mental health and well-being.
- Belonging and Becoming together foster social health and well-being.

Finally, students also explore how six pillars of health—Peace, Shelter, Education, Food and Income, Stable Ecosystems, and Equity—all depend on doing, being, becoming, and belonging or, in other words, foundational pillars of health are supported or insulted through occupation.

Through this exploration, students discover that specific occupations elicit and integrate multiple dimensions of human experience, including the following:

- Physical and biological systems
- Information processing systems
- Sociocultural contexts
- Symbolic-evaluative experience
- Transcendental experience (Sadlo, 2016)

Students must then synthesize all the above to describe how, through specific occupations, people meet primary health and well-being needs identified by occupational scientists such as the following:

- Basic survival
- Social connections
- Psychological needs for competence, autonomy, relatedness, and growth (Matuska & Christiansen, 2008)

- Unity among their bodies, minds, contexts, relationships, communities, and societies (Molineux, 2009)
- Peace, shelter, education, food, income, stable ecosystem, social justice, and equity (Wilcock & Hocking, 2015)

CONSIDER YOUR OWN TEACHING

- Do my current methods help students focus on the macro-level contexts of specific occupations?
- Do they help students understand and explain the relationships between specific occupations and the health and well-being of individuals, groups, and populations?

If the answers suggest gaps, the SCIL-OT Model encourages us to adopt highly integrative teaching and learning strategies to better facilitate the connections.

We next explore several key challenges and strategies for doing so.

Teaching Occupation: Challenges and Strategies

Challenge #1

A pervasive challenge in teaching occupation was alluded to in the earlier example of eating. The challenge is this: it is possible to teach the procedural aspects of specific occupations without addressing how and why they function as instruments of health and well-being.

To illustrate this further, consider a common topic in occupational therapy education: occupation analysis. Students who learn the procedures of occupation analysis without understanding how specific occupations support health and well-being may fail to grasp why occupation analysis is a preeminent skill in occupational therapy.

The SCIL-OT Model reminds educators to connect learning about specific occupations to the dynamics of occupation. When students learn occupation analysis in direct relation to these dynamics, they gain a deeper rationale for analyzing and adapting occupations—beyond simply improving clients' performance and engagement.

They begin to see that the occupations they analyze and adapt are part of a broader repertoire through which clients meet survival, psychological, social, spiritual, and physical needs essential to health and well-being. As a result, students learn to analyze specific occupations in ways that allow them to present and modify those occupations as levers of health and well-being (Matuska & Christiansen, 2008).

Knowing why they are learning occupation analysis empowers students to represent occupational therapy's distinct perspective and value—especially when addressing clients' most basic skills. They begin to develop literacy in occupation as humans' "primary health mechanism" (Wilcock & Hocking, 2015, p. 89).

CONSIDER YOUR OWN TEACHING

- Are students having to explain occupation as a mechanism for survival, growth, and connection?

Challenge #2

A second challenge is this: as educators, we may *overestimate students' existing knowledge* of the dynamics of occupation and their capacity to make the connections back to such dynamics from traditional learning experiences.

Because of our own experience in practice, education, and research, we as educators may assume it's self-evident how specific occupations connect to health and well-being.

But for students, these connections may remain obscure.

The SCIL-OT Model guides educators and faculty groups to

- identify specific occupations that appear in courses.
- design learning experiences that clearly and substantively include how each occupation relates to the dynamics of occupation.

Challenge #3

A third challenge relates to the *breadth of occupation*. Educators may assume that teaching the dynamics of occupation involves re-teaching content from undergraduate or prerequisite courses—such as neuroanatomy, anthropology, political science, psychology, or sociology. While students may draw on prior knowledge from these disciplines, applying it to occupation is new.

Guided by the SCIL-OT Model, educators do not re-teach prior content. Instead, we help students see occupation as something that arises from complex personal and macro-level processes—processes that together may profoundly influence a person's health and well-being.

The element of Occupation in the SCIL-OT is overall guided by this principle:

> *Occupation is the core subject of occupational therapy; therefore, occupation is the core subject of occupational therapy education.*

Second Element: Topics

The second element of the SCIL-OT Model encompasses the many important and necessary *topics* that educators teach (refer to Figure 4.1 to visualize how topics interact with all other elements in the SCIL-OT Model).

Topics are broadly defined as the explicit practice-related skills, concepts, facts, theories, attitudes, or dispositions that educators teach and students apply on a given day. This element also includes curricular threads, themes, or pillars—such as evidence-based practice, client-centered practice, or ethical practice.

At the course level, topics often appear in weekly schedules on syllabi. Examples include the following:

- Splinting
- A particular conceptual practice model
- Transfers
- Technology
- Musculoskeletal structures of the hand
- Needs assessment with community agencies

Topics are also reflected in instructional materials and in what educators explain and demonstrate to students.

The topics occupational therapy students are required to learn can feel endless.

Importantly, these topics are *not equivalent to*—nor substitutes for—the core subject of occupation. Distinguishing occupation from topics allows us to see the nature of the topics we teach in three key ways:

1. *Topics are generally not profession-specific.*
   While exceptions exist, most topics in occupational therapy curricula are not unique to the profession. Students across health disciplines learn about the following:

   - Client-centered and evidence-based practices
   - Activity analysis
   - Systems views of humans and environments
   - Anatomy, neuroscience, physiology, and psychology

2. *Topics are context-specific.*
   Practice settings, geographical regions, educational institutions, and accreditation requirements all influence which topics are taught. Topics considered essential in one program or region may be absent in another. For example:

   - One program may devote weeks to the Model of Human Occupation (MOHO; Taylor, 2017), while another may not include it at all.
   - One program may prioritize driving-related skills, while another may offer only a single lecture on the topic.

3. *Topics vary by educator.*
   Educators often teach what they have valued in their own learning and research (Lattuca & Stark, 2011). For instance:

   - An educator who had a positive experience with cadaver anatomy may believe all students should learn it in the same way.
   - Another who had an "aha" moment with emotional intelligence may seek ways to integrate it into the curriculum.
   - A researcher focused on cognitive behavioral therapy may incorporate it into their course design.

The element of Topics in the SCIL-OT is overall guided by this principle:

> *The topics we teach, although important and necessary, are not distinctive to occupational therapy and lack a cohesive logic.*

Teaching Topics: Challenges and Strategies

Challenge #1

Teaching topics is indispensable. However, their nature clarifies that topics alone do not form a cohesive professional logic. Because of this, students are unlikely to automatically see meaningful links to occupation—especially when topics are taught in a *stand-alone fashion*. As Elder and Paul (1994) noted, teaching content in isolation can leave students with a collection of unrelated bits of information that they cannot assemble or apply in profession-specific ways.

Educators are therefore challenged to teach topics in ways that:

- do not occlude occupation from students' view.
- make occupation impossible to ignore.

The SCIL-OT Model emphasizes that occupational therapy's uniqueness lies in its *core subject of occupation*—and that connection-making between topics and occupation is essential. When educators explicitly connect topics to occupation, students are most likely to grasp the distinct value of occupational therapy. Learning experiences that repeatedly, thoughtfully, and precisely draw these connections best prepare students to deliver that distinct value in practice.

Challenge #2

A related challenge is the *sheer volume* of topics educators feel compelled to teach.

Educators often begin curriculum design by asking, "*What do students need to know?*," and producing in response a list of potential topics. This question and approach reflect a *content paradigm*—an instructional design approach critiqued by Fink (2013).

In a content paradigm, educators:

- start by listing and arranging topics.
- then build courses and curricula that are *over-stuffed* with content.

This over-stuffing can obscure how topics relate to occupation—and how they relate to each other. Rather than overloading content, the SCIL-OT Model prioritizes *connection-making*:

- Connecting topics to other topics
- Connecting topics to occupation

CONSIDER YOUR OWN TEACHING

- Are students learning topics in ways that highlight their relevance to occupation?
- Are they seeing how topics interrelate, rather than treating them as isolated units?

Third Element: The Knowledge Community

Knowledge and professions are inherently *social*. They are shaped through experience, dialogue, inquiry, and discovery—processes that unfold over time through human interaction (Abbott, 2014). The SCIL-OT Model highlights this social nature by recognizing the *knowledge community* as its third element (refer to Figure 4.1 to visualize how the Knowledge Community interacts with all other elements in the SCIL-OT Model).

Members of the knowledge community may include anyone—within or outside the profession—who brings insights that illuminate the core subject of occupation and relevant topics. These insights may come from personal, practice, research, or other lived experiences.

Members can include the following:

- Educators
- Researchers
- Authors
- Interdisciplinary colleagues
- Community partners
- Vendors
- Clients and others in the client's constellation
- Students themselves

Using the SCIL-OT Model to guide curriculum and instructional design, educators intentionally create opportunities for students to *co-construct knowledge* with others. These opportunities may be

- *direct*, such as collaborating with peers in the classroom or with clients in the community.
- *indirect*, such as engaging with authors through readings or analyzing video cases.

CONSIDER YOUR OWN TEACHING

- Are students invited to see themselves as contributors to an evolving, shared body of knowledge?
- Are they learning to engage with diverse voices and perspectives around occupation-related concerns?

The element of Knowledge Community in the SCIL-OT is overall guided by this principle:

> *As members of a large knowledge community, educators and students together learn and develop knowledge of occupation and related topics.*

The Knowledge Community: Challenges and Strategies

A common challenge is that incoming students often don't realize they've joined a professional knowledge community. They may also be unaware that they're expected to be active constructors of knowledge alongside other members. To help students embrace this role, educators often design curricula that support professional socialization.

The SCIL-OT Model urges us to address socialization in *specific and explicit ways*. For example, we can intentionally design opportunities for students to connect and collaborate with the following:

- Educators
- Peers
- Clients
- Families and communities
- Interprofessional colleagues
- Organizations
- Occupational therapy practitioners and researchers

Learning activities that support these connections might include the following:

- Facilitating meetings between students and authors of their textbooks or scholarly articles
- Structuring reflections on attendance at state or national conferences
- Organizing formal and informal debates on professional issues
- Requiring students to learn about clients' lived experiences and generate implications for practice

While many programs already use such activities, the SCIL-OT Model encourages us to take them *one step further*. Students need to be able to *explicitly describe* how they are consuming and co-constructing knowledge of occupation through these collaborations.

CONSIDER YOUR OWN TEACHING

- Are students learning to articulate how their interactions shape their understanding of occupation?
- Are they being guided to see themselves as active participants in a dynamic, evolving knowledge community?

Element Four: The Learning Context

Learning context refers to the *external and internal influences* on curricula, teaching, and learning (refer to Figure 4.1 to visualize how the learning context interacts with all other elements in the SCIL-OT Model).

These influences include the following:

- New knowledge, trends, and issues in the profession
- The type and mission of the educational institution
- Geographical and cultural location
- Physical environment and available resources
- The program's vision and mission
- Faculty backgrounds, values, and teaching approaches
- Student characteristics and prior experiences

Guided by the SCIL-OT Model, educators seek to recognize how these contextual influences shape

- how occupation is understood.
- which occupations are deemed most relevant.
- which topics are prioritized.
- who comprises the knowledge community.
- which teaching methods are most valued.

Careful attention to these influences helps students understand why learners in other programs may have *very different educational experiences*. For example:

- In a program committed to *problem-based learning*, students' experiences will be shaped by how cases are designed, tutors are trained, and debriefings are conducted.

- In a program with resources for *standardized patients*, students' learning will depend on how actors are trained, what students are asked to do, and the feedback they receive.
- In a school with a strong *interprofessional education initiative*, students will engage in articulating occupational therapy's distinct value in specific client situations.

The element of Learning Context in the SCIL-OT is overall guided by this principle:

> *The learning context of the specific program shapes all elements of the SCIL-OT model for that program.*

The Learning Context: Challenges and Strategies

Given the wide range of possible contextual influences, a common challenge is discerning which influences to assess in order to illuminate constraints and opportunities for curriculum and instructional design.

Fink (2013) and Lattuca and Stark (2011) recommend assessing the following:

- Trends in the profession and marketplace
- Institutional type and priorities
- Program and faculty characteristics
- Learner characteristics
- Curriculum sequence
- Learning resources

These areas of assessment align with the SCIL-OT Model's emphasis on learning context. However, the SCIL-OT Model further specifies *unique features* to consider:

Educators are urged to assess

- how the collective *occupational profile* of students in a program should influence teaching and learning.
- whether occupations characteristic of the campus, community, or region can be used to teach the dynamics of occupation.
- whether existing programs offer opportunities for students to hone an occupational perspective.
- what ongoing occupational needs exist in the campus, community, or region—and how students might learn about and address those needs.

- the extent to which faculty are well versed in an occupational view of humans and the dynamics of occupation—and related opportunities for faculty development.

CONSIDER YOUR OWN PROGRAM

- What contextual influences most shape your curriculum?
- How might you leverage local occupations or community needs to deepen students' understanding of occupation?

Element Five: The Connecting Lines

The fifth element of the SCIL-OT Model consists of the *lines that interconnect* all other elements. Designing curricula and instruction *on-the-lines* is the principle that brings *subject-centered integrative learning* to life.

Learning on-the-lines means designing instruction that shifts students' attention away from isolated topics, experiences, and interactions—and toward five key connections:

- Specific occupations to the dynamics of occupation
- Topics to the core subject of occupation
- Various topics to one another
- Students' experiences to the core subject of occupation
- Students to members of knowledge communities in their given contexts

CONSIDER YOUR OWN TEACHING:

- Are students being guided to make these five connections regularly and explicitly?
- How might your instructional design better support connection-making?

To support these connections, the SCIL-OT Model aligns well with many *common teaching and assessment methods*.

Educators frequently

- set up active learning experiences in classrooms and communities.
- demonstrate, model, lecture, and facilitate discussion.

- use electronic materials, ask questions, and give feedback.
- provide physical and visual prompts.

They also incorporate

- interprofessional experiences.
- team- and problem-based cases.
- standardized patient encounters.
- simulation-based learning.

Assessment methods often include

- written examinations.
- treatment plans.
- client presentations.
- practical examinations.

Guided by the SCIL-OT Model, educators continue to use these methods—but with a *critical redirection*: Instructional design, teaching methods, and learning outcomes are aimed *directly at students' connection-making* across the five dimensions listed earlier.

CONSIDER YOUR OWN PROGRAM

- Are your assessments helping students demonstrate how they connect topics to occupation?
- Are your learning activities structured to reveal the integrative nature of occupational therapy?

The element of Learning-on-the-Lines in the SCIL-OT is overall guided by this principle:

> *Teaching, learning, and assessment occur 'on-the-lines' between the model's elements, representing a continuous process of knowledge co-creation.*

Connections of Topics to the Core Subject of Occupation: Challenges and Strategies

To ensure students develop a deep knowledge of occupation—and the ability to use it therapeutically—the SCIL-OT Model reminds educators that *all topics* must be related not only to specific occupations but also to *why and how* those occupations function as mechanisms of health and well-being.

Rather than teaching topics in a stand-alone fashion, we teach the relationships between topics, specific occupations, and the dynamics of occupation.

Topics relate to occupation in several ways. A topic may

- develop through occupation (e.g., skills and capacities).
- thwart occupation (e.g., poverty or disability).
- enable occupation directly, without therapist involvement (e.g., humans' need and drive for occupation).
- serve as a tool therapists use to enable occupation (e.g., client-centered practice, therapeutic use of self).
- provide a way of conceptualizing occupation and its relation to health and well-being (e.g., MOHO).
- be a facet of occupation (e.g., meaning).
- support therapists in enabling occupation (e.g., knowledge of health disparities, leadership).

We may teach these relationships through problem-based learning, lecture, discussion, service learning, or other methods. Regardless of method, the *instructional target* is students' ability to connect topics to occupation—that is, their *on-the-line knowledge*.

We also assess this knowledge by designing exams, essays, intervention plans, documentation assignments, or other assessments that evaluate not only the topic itself but also the *strength and clarity of the connections* students draw to the core of the profession.

Take the topic of anatomy or kinesiology, for example.

Teaching on-the-lines means that beyond learning musculoskeletal structures and functions, students learn to connect those structures and functions to *the performance of specific occupations*.

Going further, students learn to connect movement—its type, extent, and intensity—to

- environmental transactions.
- intentions and biological conditions (e.g., hunger and fatigue).
- demands of the occupation.

- meaning, volition, and cognition.

In other words, students learn body functions and structures in connection to the mechanisms that make occupation an agent of health and well-being, as described in Chapter 2.

When guided by the SCIL-OT Model, educators ask the following:

- What are the relationships between each topic in this course and specific occupations and the dynamics of occupation?
- How will my instructional design help students make these connections?
- How will my assessment strategies ensure students can demonstrate these connections?

CONSIDER YOUR OWN TEACHING

- Are students learning to see topics as tools for understanding and enabling occupation?
- Are your assessments designed to reveal students' integrative thinking

Connections Among Various Topics: Challenges and Strategies

Occupational therapy educators are often *highly skilled* at designing activities that require students to integrate multiple topics. Activities related to the *occupational therapy process* are prime examples. We commonly ask students to

- interview people about their occupational histories, current challenges, and perceived strengths.
- observe an occupation.
- assess and document occupational strengths and challenges.
- draft goals to address those challenges.
- plan and sometimes implement an intervention.

We also frequently require students to

- connect topics to supporting research.
- apply theoretical concepts to practice.

When we assign these activities, we are asking students to interconnect knowledge of

- occupation.
- the occupational therapy process.
- interpersonal and communication skills.
- interviewing.
- documentation and other topics.

However, we *less commonly ask students to identify explicitly* which topics they had to integrate to complete an activity (Hooper et al., 2018). Without this step, students may not develop metacognitive awareness of how they assemble and draw upon distinct knowledge domains. As a result, the broader conceptual understandings needed to complete the activity may remain *veiled*, leaving students unaware of how they construct knowledge for practice.

To fully support integration, educators must take one additional step:

Ask students to identify the topics they combined and explain how each informed their performance. For example, when planning an intervention, a small group of students might identify the topics they assembled:

- They begin with *interviewing skills* to elicit the client's occupational goals and discover a desire to cook a simple meal.
- They link this to knowledge of *roles and role fulfillment* to highlight the occupation's importance.
- They use *observation skills* and *occupation analysis* to assess the fit between the client's capacities, kitchen environment, and cooking task.
- They combine observation with *motor assessments* based on what they observed.
- They apply knowledge of *object characteristics* to select tools and materials that are not too heavy.
- They draw on *person-environment-occupation alignment* to position tools and materials, mindful of reduced range of motion.
- Throughout, they use *client-centered care* to engage the client in collaborative problem solving.

When guided by the SCIL-OT Model, educators ask:

- How do the topics in my course connect to each other?
- How can I design instruction to help students make those connections?

- Do my learning activities and assessments hold students accountable for connecting topics?
- Have I asked students to identify the topics they assembled to complete the activity or assessment?

CONSIDER YOUR OWN TEACHING

- Are students aware of the knowledge domains they're integrating?
- Are you helping them name and explain those connections?

Connections of Students' Own Life Experiences to the Dynamics of Occupation: Challenges and Strategies

Occupational therapy educators are also masterful at teaching *on-the-lines* between students and occupation. A common assignment across programs involves asking students to complete time use diaries and analyze them for types, patterns, and routines of occupation.

Students may also

- analyze an occupation and its role in shaping their development, identity, capacities, meaning system, and time use.
- reflect on the loss of a favored occupation and its impact on self, habits, routines, and capacities.
- learn a new occupation and discuss what it brought to their lives, including an analysis of its demands.

In these and similar activities, we ask students to connect with occupation on a *personal level*.

This personal connection shifts occupation from something 'out there' to something students can relate to, see as relevant, and ultimately with careful knowledge translation strategies apply to their understanding with clients.

However, we can take these analyses one step further to deepen students' understanding of the mechanisms by which occupation influences health and well-being. Sometimes, students complete insightful personal analyses—but the activity ends there.

To fully realize the learning potential, students must also grasp the *macro-level occupation–health dynamics* illustrated in their own experiences.

When guided by the SCIL-OT Model, educators ask:

- Is there an opportunity in my course for students to relate personally to the concept of occupation?
- When students examine occupation in their own lives, have I asked them to link it to the *macro influences* that made those occupations possible—or that disrupted them?
- Have I asked students to trace the impact of occupation all the way to their *health, well-being, development, and retention of capacities*?
- Have I asked students to summarize *why occupation is occupational therapy's central concern*, based on their personal experiences?

CONSIDER YOUR OWN TEACHING

- Are students learning to see their own lives as evidence of occupation's therapeutic power?
- Are they being guided to connect personal insight with professional understanding?

Connections with Members of the Knowledge Community in Given Learning Contexts: Challenges and Strategies

Occupational therapy educators commonly teach *on-the-lines* between students and other members of the knowledge community—though we seldom frame it this way. For example:

- When we ask students to read scholarly literature, we are guiding them to connect with authors as members of the knowledge community.
- When students interview people, engage with guest lecturers, or participate in peer discussions, they are connecting with others whose experiences and insights shape their understanding of occupation and related topics.

In these interactions, students are asked to

- inquire.
- critically evaluate.
- take in personal experiences and scholarship.

These connections support students in *constructing knowledge*, not just receiving it.

What we often omit, however, is an explicit expectation that students recognize and name their own knowledge-making process through these engagements.

Students may not realize

- how they are assembling knowledge from others into a personal knowledge base.
- how they are actively changing their thinking in response to new insights.
- how they are revising the meaning of prior experiences based on new learning.

Teaching *on-the-lines* among the knowledge community means creating opportunities for students to see themselves as:

- *Receiving knowledge* from others
- *Co-creating knowledge* with others

We design learning so that students can *see and describe* the active knowledge creation they do in response to interactions with readings (authors), guests, interviewees, and peers.

When guided by the SCIL-OT Model, educators ask:

- What members of the knowledge community are relevant to my course?
- How will students connect with those identified members?
- Toward what learning outcomes will students' connections contribute?
- How will students explain the knowledge they created in collaboration with members of the knowledge community?

CONSIDER YOUR OWN TEACHING

- Are students being guided to reflect on how their thinking evolves through engagement with others?
- Are they learning to see themselves as contributors to a shared professional knowledge base?

SUMMARY AND CONCLUSION

Nearly two decades ago, Whiteford and Wilcock (2001) identified a persistent shortfall in occupational therapy education:

> *[I]n the minds of students who have no clear notion of why they are learning anatomy, physiology or neuroscience and how these subjects contribute to the occupational therapy profession's particular view of humans, such subjects can become ends in themselves. This is particularly compounded when such topics . . . are delivered without an appropriate orientation as to why, and to what extent, occupational therapists need to understand the material covered. When this is the case, it is not surprising that students of occupational therapy struggle to integrate such knowledge into an understanding of occupation and applied occupational therapy concepts.*
>
> (p. 82)

The struggle to integrate knowledge of occupation with other topics is particularly concerning. Integration is, after all, an essential quality of knowledge in occupational therapy (Hooper & Wood, 2018). Moreover, multiple professions—including medicine, nursing, and engineering—have identified similar insufficiencies resulting from teaching topics in stand-alone fashions.

To address these gaps, these professions have initiated reforms toward integrative, subject-centered learning. Grounded in occupation and focused on connection-making across knowledge domains, the SCIL-OT Model offers a pathway for occupational therapy educators to do the same.

The model is built on the principle that the big ideas of occupational therapy must also be the big ideas of occupational therapy education.

These big ideas are informed by the core subject of occupation:

- That humans meet needs for survival and thriving through occupations coordinated with other occupations.
- That occupations manifest deeper mechanisms affecting health and well-being—sustaining transactions among biological needs, contexts, time, habits, and culture.

In other words, the dynamics of occupation.

The model also recognizes that teaching topics is vital. Yet when topics and skills are taught apart from these big ideas, students may struggle to apply the logic of their profession in practice.

Additionally, the SCIL-OT Model is guided by learning principles that emphasize:

- students' roles as active knowledge-creators in learning communities.
- the importance of situating curricula and the concept of occupation in local contexts and communities.

Most importantly, the SCIL-OT Model encourages educators to teach—and students to learn—how to draw *myriad connections* between the profession's core subject of occupation and the *diverse topics and domains of knowledge* that occupational therapy practice demands.

CONSIDER YOUR OWN CURRICULUM

- Are the big ideas of occupational therapy clearly visible in your teaching?
- Are students learning to integrate knowledge in ways that reflect the profession's logic and values?

REFERENCES

Abbott, A. (2014). *The system of professions: An essay on the division of expert labor*. University of Chicago Press.

American Occupational Therapy Association. (2020). *Occuaptional Therapy Practice Framework: Domain and process* (4th ed.). Author.

Bagatell, N., & Womack, J. L. (2016). Human capacity for action as core content in occupational science education. *Journal of Occupational Science*, *23*(4), 514–518. https://doi.org/10.1080/14427591.2016.1226682

Elder, L., & Paul, R. (1994). Critical thinking: Why we must transform our teaching. *Journal of Developmental Education*, *18*(1), 34–35.

Fink, L. (2013). *Creating significant learning experiences: An integrated approach to designing college courses*. Jossey-Bass.

Fisher, A., & Marterella, A. (2019). *Powerful practice: A model for authentic occupational therapy*. Center for Innovative OT Solutions.

Hooper, B., & Wood, W. (2018). The philosophy of occupational therapy: A framework for practice. In B. Schell, G. Gillen, & M. Scaffa (Eds.), *Willard & Spackman's occupational therapy* (12th ed., pp. 5–46). Wolters Kluwer.

Hooper, B., Krishnagiri, S., Price, P., Taff, S., & Bilics, A. (2018). Curriculum-level strategies that U.S. occupational therapy programs use to address occupation: A qualitative study. *American Journal of Occupational Therapy*, *72*(1), 7201205040p7201205041–7201205040p7201205010.

Lattuca, L., & Stark, J. (2011). *Shaping the college curriculum: Academic plans in context* (2nd ed.). Jossey-Bass.

Matuska, K., & Christiansen, C. (2008). A proposed model of lifestyle balance. *Journal of Occupational Science*, *15*(1), 9–19.

Molineux, M. (2009). The nature of occupation. In M. Curtin, M. Molineux, & J. Supyk-Mellson (Eds.), *Occupational therapy and physical dysfunction: Enabling occupation* (6th ed., pp. 17–26). Elsevier.

Sadlo, G. (2016). Threshold concepts for educating people about human engagement in occupation: The study of human systems that enable occupation. *Journal of Occupational Science*, *23*(4), 496–509.

Taylor, R. (Ed.). (2017). *Kielhofner's model of human occupation: Theory and application* (5th ed.). Lippincott Williams & Wilkins.

Townsend, E., & Polatajko, H. (Eds.). (2013). *Enabling occupation II: Advancing an occupational therapy vision for health, well-being, & justice through occupation* (2nd ed.). Canadian Association of Occupational Therapists.

Whiteford, G., & Wilcock, A. (2001). Centralizing occupation in occupational therapy curricula: Imperative of the new millennium. *Occupational Therapy International*, *8*(2), 81–85.

Wilcock, A., & Hocking, C. (2015). *An occupational perspective of health* (3rd ed.). Slack.

Part II

Applying the SCIL-OT Model Across the Curriculum

Part II translates the SCIL-OT Model into practice. Annotated examples, design prompts, and practical strategies guide educators in transforming curriculum documents, course descriptions and structure, classroom activities, learning, assessment, and practice education to make occupation visible, connected, and central across all levels of a curriculum.

DOI: 10.4324/9781003635628-6

Chapter 5

Connecting Student Learning to Occupation

INTRODUCTION

This chapter is a first in a series of chapters that elaborate on, provide examples of, and offer design activities for each element of the SCIL-OT model introduced in Chapter 4. This chapter addresses and further elucidates the core element of the model, which is occupation. Occupation is the defining feature of occupational therapy because it captures our unique perspective of humans and health and well-being. Occupation is, therefore, at the heart of the SCIL-OT Model in order to demonstrate the centrality of occupation to all aspects of occupational therapy education. The model portrays occupation as having two dimensions to consider when designing learning experiences, specific occupations and the dynamics of occupation. Encompassing these two dimensions, occupation serves as the big idea of the field and as the organizing framework for education, against which other content can be positioned for learners (Hansen, 2011; Wiggins & McTighe, 2011).

While it is beyond the scope of this chapter to address all knowledge, skills, and attitudes associated with learning about occupation and its relationship with health and well-being, we encourage educators to reflect on the material covered and to undertake the informal self-assessment from Chapter 2 of your own expertise in relation to occupation and its relationship with health and well-being.

OBJECTIVES

This chapter will help educators to:

1. Design learning opportunities that help students understand occupation as the core across the four component areas of a curriculum: the education program, the courses, the classroom, and practice education.

DOI: 10.4324/9781003635628-7

2. Assess and strengthen the focus on occupation across the four component areas of a curriculum.

OCCUPATION: THE PROFESSION'S CORE SUBJECT

As outlined in Chapter 4, the view taken by us, which is supported by educational theory and research, is that in order to design effective entry level educational experiences for students, educators must recognize that the core of the profession is occupation. As such educators must be knowledgeable about, and skilled in our use of, occupation, but we must also be deliberate and explicit in linking what is taught in educational programs to occupation as the core subject of the profession.

The centrality of occupation to occupational therapy education is not new. Yerxa (1998, p. 355) argued that "occupation needs to become the central organising framework" for occupational therapy curricula, because it is occupation that differentiates our profession from others. It is the case however, that just as the centrality of occupation in the profession's philosophy and practice has waxed and waned over the years (Kielhofner, 2009) so too has its place in occupational therapy education.

The SCIL-OT Model (Figure 5.1) clearly locates occupation as the central element in education. All other elements must be explicitly linked to occupation in order for students to integrate their knowledge of topics and their interactions with the knowledge community to occupation across their educational experiences.

Due to the inherent complexity of occupation, the SCIL-OT Model includes two aspects of occupation that need to be considered when designing and delivering occupational therapy education: specific occupations and the dynamics of occupation. The core of the SCIL-OT, occupation, was outlined in Chapters 3 and 4 and in order to now consider its application in educational practice, it is important to review two key considerations.

Specific Occupations—Important but Insufficient

First, while specific occupations are easily identified by students as dressing, cooking, playing with children, driving, shopping, and so on, merely naming them does not capture the complexity of the factors and circumstance that give rise to each of those specific occupations. Similarly, students could also categorize occupations according to one of many of the taxonomies published and while that would add one piece of extra information, namely a short cut to the purpose of the occupation (e.g., self-care, productivity, leisure), it too falls short of capturing any occupation's complexity (Molineux, 2009). Students can

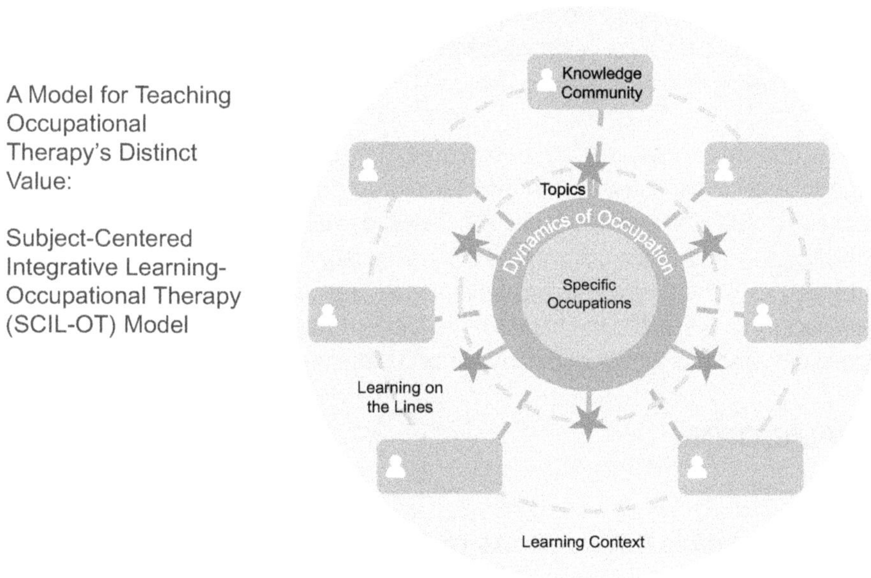

Figure 5.1 Occupation and its role in health and well-being are the organizing concept for occupational therapy education.

go another step further and analyze an occupation using other aspects of any of those taxonomies. In doing so, students will recognize the multitude of person and environment factors that enable and inhibit occupational performance and engagement including social stigma, political change, accessibility, range of motion, strength, and memory, for example. While this deepens students' understanding even more, it still falls short of a comprehensive understanding.

Dynamics of Occupation—The Complexity of Occupation and Health and Well-Being

Occupational scientists and occupational therapists have spent decades exploring the nature and inner workings of occupation and the occupation–health–well-being relationship. Though there is still much more to know, there is already, as discussed in Chapter 2, a large knowledge base to draw upon. There are, therefore, two challenges for occupational therapy educators.

First, we must achieve a high degree of familiarity with the existing and emerging theory and research on occupation and its relationship with health and well-being. Indeed, research with international experts in occupational therapy education highlighted the need for educators to be experts in the occupation–health–well-being dynamic (Canty et al., 2020). However, educators with only minimum exposure to this dynamic are still capable of designing learning in their areas of expertise that keep students making connections to occupation.

The second challenge is that we must ensure that students graduate with a sophisticated, albeit entry-level, knowledge of occupation and the relationship between occupation and health and well-being, as well as skills in applying this knowledge to individuals, communities, and populations in a range of practice settings. This is the only way to ensure that graduates can fulfill their contract with society as presented in Chapter 2—students must graduate as experts in occupation and the relationship between occupation and health and well-being.

APPLICATION

Making Explicit Connections to Occupation at the Program Level

Accreditation standards in most all jurisdictions require documents that outline the key elements of the program's curriculum design. Often these include a vision, mission, aim, philosophy, curriculum threads, and program outcomes. Occupation is core to occupational therapy, so it should feature prominently in program-level documents to signal to students and stakeholders the centrality of the concept to the profession and therefore the program. Where possible, careful attention should be given to capturing the full dynamics of occupation—specific occupations, the complex mechanisms of occupation, and the relationship between occupation and health and well-being—in program documentation. There are a number of forms this could take; for example,

- The program's philosophy could capture an overview of the history of occupational therapy in the context in which the program is located (educational institution, state/region, country) as well as the history of the profession.

BOX 5.1 SAMPLE OUTLINE OF HISTORICAL CONTENT THAT MAY APPEAR IN A PROGRAM PHILOSOPHY TO HIGHLIGHT OCCUPATION'S EVOLUTION, PROMINENCE, AND LINK TO THE PROGRAM'S IDENTITY

A program philosophy or other key program-level document may

- *recognize the historical importance of occupation* in the founding of the occupational therapy profession, while acknowledging that its centrality has fluctuated over time.

- *emphasize the contemporary renaissance of occupation* within the profession. This resurgence may be reflected in the inclusion of occupational science courses or in the integration of occupational science concepts across the curriculum.
- *identify other historically significant aspects of the profession* that are relevant to the program's identity—such as the importance of research and evidence-based practice, or the expansion of occupational therapy into non-traditional settings. These elements may serve as points of differentiation for the program.

- Program documents may describe the specific occupations, occupational patterns, occupational issues, and the dynamics of occupation most relevant in the local area. This signals to students, faculty, and stakeholders an occupational perspective of life in the local area, including the opportunities for and barriers to occupational engagement.
- The program may create a definition of occupational therapy that reflects the local history and context of the program or adopt one that exists elsewhere such as that published by World Federation of Occupational Therapists (2012) (see Box 5.1). Creating or adopting a clear definition of occupational therapy will provide an easily accessible summary of the scope of the profession and may highlight seemingly subtle but important distinctions. For example, a program that adopts a definition of occupational therapy focused on 'working with people with range of physical and mental impairments' will look different from a program that defines occupational therapy as a profession 'which seeks to promote occupational justice for all members of society.'
- Discussion of how the local context and nature of occupational therapy sit within the international occupational therapy landscape. For example, describing the extent to which local occupational therapy practice is occupation centered or biomedically focused, is located in traditional or innovative practice settings, and is located in government or non-government organizations/sectors will convey the opportunities for occupational therapy practice and the potential contextual barriers to the scope of practice.
- Specification of the knowledge, skills, and attitudes required for the particular type of occupational therapy practice outlined in the curricular documents ensuring that the dynamics of occupation are explicit.
- Program learning outcomes are another important place to demonstrate the centrality of occupation to what students will learn.
- A program aim is a succinct way to summarize the essence of the program's focus.

Table 5.1 Definition of occupational therapy (World Federation of Occupational Therapists, 2012) annotated to illustrate making occupation explicit in program-level documents.

World Federation of Occupational Therapists Definition of Occupational Therapy:	
Occupational therapy is a client-centred health profession concerned with promoting health and well-being through occupation. The primary goal of occupational therapy is to enable people to participate in the activities of everyday life... Occupational therapists achieve this outcome by working with people and communities to enhance their ability to engage... in the occupations they want to, need to, or are expected to do, ... or by modifying the occupation... or the environment to better... support their occupational engagement	◄ Link between occupation and health explicitly noted (dynamics) ◄ Specific occupations – although this definition includes only one category to capture the pervasive nature of occupation in everyday life ◄ Dynamics - person factors influence occupation ◄ Dynamics – social environment influences occupation ◄ Modifying the [specific] occupation ◄ Dynamics of occupation – environment factors influence occupation

Overall, the WFOT definition could be strengthened by elaborating on the relationship between occupation, occupational engagement, and health. A faculty group could choose to elaborate and adopt the modified definition as their guiding definition.

In addition to a program's selected definition of occupational therapy, writing the program's aim is another opportunity to emphasize occupation in a key curricular document. Tables 5.2 and 5.3 present two program aims to illustrate.

At every step of the way in developing or revising an occupational therapy program—occupation can be more or less present and explicit. Ensuring occupation is as explicit as possible in these documents lays a strong and important foundation for the outcomes, assessment plan, and courses that follow. It is probably the case

Table 5.2 Program aim annotated to illustrate how occupation can become obscured in key program-level documents.

Example Aim from Program A	
The overall aim of the program in Occupational Therapy is to provide the student with an excellent educational experience in the academic and practice environments. Successful completion of the program will enable the graduate to apply for registration with the local registration body for occupational therapists.	≺ Aim emphasizes regulatory outcomes.
The newly qualified occupational therapist will be equipped with knowledge, skills, and attributes required to work and develop as a competent practitioner within the changing health and social care environment.	≺ Profession specific practice sentence but even this is quite generic—being competent to work as an occupational therapist in appropriate environments.
However, graduating with this graduate degree will also provide the practitioner with clinical scholarship, research skills, an advanced understanding of evidence-based practice as well as leadership and innovation skills.	≺ These outcomes are not profession specific. ≺ Overall, the aim does not make explicit that occupation is at the core of the educational program.

Table 5.3 Program aim annotated to illustrate how occupation can be explicit in key program-level documents.

Example Aim from Program B	
The program aims to enable students to become occupation-centered, theory-driven, evidence-based and client-centered occupational therapists,	≺ Occupation-centered is positioned as the first, most important, characteristic of graduates from the program.
able to practice in current, emerging and future settings and roles, to enhance the health and well-being of individuals, communities and populations through occupation.	≺ Captures the dynamics of occupation—link between occupation and health and well-being. ≺ The ultimate aim of the occupational therapy services is to enhance health and well-being, and that is achieved through use of the profession's unique focus on occupation.

that sometimes these program documents are completed only for the purpose of institutional approval and accreditation purposes, and therefore once the documents have been approved, they are seldom referred to again. This is, however, a mistake as these documents form the conceptual and values base of the educational program. They should be seen as the template, a touchstone, or a check point for every step of curriculum design, delivery and evaluation, staff/faculty recruitment, student recruitment, and program development. They should also be seen as communiques to students about the specific nature of their learning.

PROGRAM LEARNING OUTCOMES

Occupational therapy education programs in most regions must identify desired student outcomes by graduation. Outcomes are another opportunity to communicate that learning in the program targets knowledge, skills, and attitudes related to occupation as a source of health and well-being. Consider, for example, the program-level learning outcomes from one undergraduate four-year bachelor program:

On successful completion of the bachelor program, students will:

- have current and in-depth knowledge of concepts and theories of relevant biomedical and health sciences.
- communicate effectively with individuals, groups and larger populations using written, spoken and technological modes.

- demonstrate commitment to lifelong learning in personal and/or professional development with a focus on innovation.
- demonstrate a commitment to ethical action and social responsibility as occupational therapy professionals.
- competently apply a professional, evidence-based, body of knowledge and high-level skills to provide safe and ethical practice.

While all of these learning outcomes are entirely reasonable and we would expect students from all occupational therapy programs to have these attributes, as written they are generic (except for naming occupational therapy in the fourth statement) and could apply to many health programs. Occupation is not made explicit—neither specific occupations nor the dynamics of occupation.

Another four-year undergraduate bachelor program uses the five curriculum areas of knowledge, skills, and attitudes for competent practice from the World Federation of Occupational Therapists (2016), that is, person–occupation–environment relationship and health and well-being, therapeutic and professional relationships, occupational therapy process, professional reasoning and behavior, and context of practice (Table 5.4). They are, therefore, more detailed, but even consideration of two of

Table 5.4 Sample program learning outcomes illustrating using World Federation of Occupational Therapists' (2016) five curriculum areas to center knowledge and skills focused on occupation.

WFOT curriculum area: Person–occupation–environment relationship and health		
Type of outcome	**Related program outcomes**	
Knowledge	Appraise health and well-being from an occupational perspective.	◀ Names the profession's unique perspective on humans and health.
	Critique the relationship between occupational performance and engagement and participation.	◀ Explicitly identifies occupation, health, and participation in all learning outcomes.
Skill	Create interventions to optimize occupational performance and engagement, and participation.	◀ Clarifies that occupation and health are the focus of assessment and intervention.

Table 5.4 (Continued)

	WFOT curriculum area: Context of practice	
Knowledge	Interpret current, emerging, and future contexts of occupational therapy practice.	◀ Highlights that there are multiple contexts/environments that enable/inhibit occupational performance and engagement, without limiting that list of contexts that might be relevant to the profession.
Skill	Hypothesize about how an occupational perspective can inform local and global health and well-being issues.	◀ Makes explicit that an occupational perspective can add value to all health issues.

those areas shows that, at the program-level, occupation is explicit in the outcomes. Although occupation is explicit, specific occupations and the dynamics of occupation are less explicit but can be implied.

Making occupation explicit in program-level outcomes is particularly important because outcomes drive program assessment. Well-crafted outcomes will help ensure that the program measures how well students master learning and practice skills related to improving health through occupation.

MAKING EXPLICIT CONNECTIONS TO OCCUPATION AT THE COURSE LEVEL

There are multiple opportunities to make occupation explicit to students at the course level of the program. We highlight three here: course titles, course descriptions, and the course schedule.

Course Titles and Descriptions

The names that courses are given and the descriptions that appear online are often the first place that students encounter a course and so the messages conveyed in these brief statements set the scene and sensitize students to what is important and what is not important in that course. Consider the two courses in Table 5.5.

Table 5.5 Course titles and descriptions illustrating varying emphasis on occupation.

Example Course Description A (taught within the OT program):	
OCT999—Functional Anatomy for Occupational Therapy	◄ Course title does not reference occupation
An overview of human anatomy for occupational therapy students . . .	◄ States the course is specific to "occupational therapy students" but does not reference occupation, occupational performance, or engagement.
. . including musculoskeletal, nervous, cardiovascular, respiratory, digestive and urinary systems.	◄ Captures the topics but not how the topics of this course link to the core subject of the profession.
Example Course Description B (taught within the OT program):	
OCT999—Human Capacities: Body Structures and Functions 1	◄ This course does not include a link to occupation in the title but Human Capacities implies something beyond structures alone.
This course provides an introduction to the structures, functions, and processes of the human body that support participation in occupation.	◄ Identifies for students the link between "structures, functions, and processes of the human body" to the their relevance for occupational therapy—participation in occupation.
The course will focus on mental processes, sensory processing, digestion, reproduction, endocrine, and immune responses that support human occupation.	◄ Specific topics or content areas are left to the final sentence and again link to their relevance tohuman occupation

Course Schedule in the Syllabus

In addition to course titles and descriptions, how the sequence of a course is represented can also focus students' attention on what is most important. The course sequence is often a schedule of the days the course meets and what topics will be addressed on each day. Consider the first six weeks of two syllabi for a course called Pediatric Dysfunction and Occupation (Table 5.6) The course overview states that the course focuses on conditions commonly encountered by occupational therapists including knowledge of conditions and the impact of those conditions on occupation.

At one level, the topics in Table 5.6, Course A, are completely appropriate for a course that seeks to introduce students to a range of diagnoses. However, occupation remains hidden from students in this topic overview. Not apparent in this sequence are

- the specific occupations of childhood.
- the dynamics of occupation.
- how and why the occupations associated with studying at school—getting to/from school, participating in classes, attending the prom, toileting, buying and eating lunch etc.—are impacted (or not) by the person factors associated with a condition, or the complex interaction between the person factors of the condition, the physical and social environments, and occupations.
- how all of these issues impact on the health and well-being of children, their families, their school, and the wider community.

Table 5.6 Course syllabus topics for two courses on Pediatric Dysfunction and Occupation illustrating varying emphasis on occupation.

Week	Sequence of topics: illustration from Course A	Sequence of topics: illustration from Course B
1	Course introduction Premature and high-risk infants	Course introduction Children as occupational beings
2	OT Practice Framework Neural tube defects Cerebral palsy	Occupational development
3	Cerebral palsy continued Traumatic brain injury Epilepsy	Self-care occupations
4	Neuromuscular disorders Musculoskeletal disorders Orthopedic conditions	Productivity occupations
5	Vision Hearing Sensory processing disorders	Leisure occupations
5	Intellectual disabilities Down syndrome Fetal alcohol syndrome	Children's occupations in the context of family

We recognize that a published sequence may not fully capture the breadth of topics addressed in a day. It is possible, however, to craft the course schedule in ways that capture clearly the "why" of the learning in addition to specific topics.

An occupation-centered course syllabus might first consider child development from an occupational perspective (Humphry & Wakeford, 2005) and contrast this with the dominant perspectives of child development from psychology such as cognitive theories, psychosexual theories, social learning theories, or behavioral theories. The revised topics might look like those presented in Table 5.6, Course B.

Note that while not prioritized or privileged in the course syllabus, the course instructor could incorporate a range of conditions and consider them in relation to the focus for that week. For example, when focusing on children as occupational beings one subtopic might be children who are born prematurely and/or with congenital impairments and how their occupational development is impacted from birth. When considering self-care occupations, the instructor might use spina bifida as an example of how person factors such as incontinence impact on the child's engagement in occupations such as toileting; for example, the child may require assistance with toileting until they are older compared with a child without spina bifida. The classes on productivity occupations might focus exclusively on education settings and consider how a child with an eating disorder might have particular challenges with the occupations usually engaged in while at school.

MAKING EXPLICIT CONNECTIONS TO OCCUPATION AT THE CLASSROOM LEVEL

One common classroom activity used to explore occupation is the time use diary. Students are typically asked to record what they do each hour for a week. Depending on the learning objectives, instructions may vary—from 'document everything you do' to 'record the occupations you engaged in'.

This activity can be a powerful tool for teaching about occupation—but its impact depends on how it is used. A basic analysis might ask students to:

- list all the specific occupations they engaged in.
- categorize those occupations using a framework.

This can help students recognize:

- the richness of daily life, by counting the number and variety of occupations.
- differences in categorization, such as one student labeling cooking breakfast as self-care, while another sees it as productivity.

To deepen learning using the SCIL-OT Model, educators can additionally guide students to explore the dynamics of occupation. For example:

Ask students to pair up and compare similar occupations from their diaries (e.g., showering or cooking breakfast). Have them describe what they did and reflect on differences in the following:

- Personal meaning
- Cultural significance
- Physical environment
- Health and well-being transaction
- Time of day
- Personal preferences
- Occupational history

This approach helps students see that even when occupations appear similar, their dynamics vary widely. It reinforces the idea that occupation is not just what people do—but how, why, and under what conditions they do it.

By making these dynamics explicit, educators help students build a more nuanced understanding of occupation—and prepare them to apply this understanding in practice.

MAKING EXPLICIT CONNECTIONS TO OCCUPATION IN PRACTICE EDUCATION

In practice education, students can sometimes lose sight of occupation. As they enter unfamiliar settings—such as hospitals or correctional facilities—they often focus their energy on learning about the population, the setting, or the knowledge community. In the process, the core of occupation may fade into the background.

The SCIL-OT Model can help students stay anchored in the profession's core. One simple strategy is to ask students to use an occupational therapy conceptual model to analyze a client's occupational performance and engagement. This reminds them that even when the setting is new, their role is to understand the person as an occupational being—and to explore how occupation supports health and well-being (see Chapparo et al., 2017).

For example, a student working with someone recently released from prison might be overwhelmed by the legal and social context. But those factors only become relevant to occupational therapy when they help us understand how the person engages in occupation—and how that engagement supports or hinders health.

Students can be asked to complete a written or oral occupation analysis using a recognized model. This could be shared with their supervisor, the occupational therapy department, or the interdisciplinary team. However, it's important that the analysis:

- goes beyond naming or categorizing person, environment, and occupation factors.
- addresses the dynamic transactions between these elements.
- explores how those transactions relate to health and well-being.

Role-emerging placements—where there is no established occupational therapy role—offer both a challenge and an opportunity.

- The challenge is staying grounded in occupation without the structure of traditional practice.
- The opportunity is the freedom to define the role from an occupation-centered perspective.

To support students in these settings, educators can introduce an occupation-centered process model such as the Canadian Practice Process Framework (CPPF) (Craik et al., 2013; Davis et al., 2013). This model keeps occupation central throughout the process. For example:

- *Stage 2* ends with collaboratively identifying occupational issues—not just problems or symptoms.
- *Stage 3* involves identifying barriers and enablers to occupational performance and engagement.
- *Stage 4* focuses on setting occupational goals and planning interventions.
- *Stage 5* involves engaging the client in occupation as part of the intervention.

Students can use the process model before they work with a client and anticipate actions associated with each stage. Or they can review a client case retroactively to identify the actions associated with each stage and what they overlooked or where they could strengthen going forward. By following a process that centers occupation, students are better equipped to contribute meaningfully—even in unfamiliar or emerging practice settings.

ASSESSING STUDENTS' UNDERSTANDINGS OF OCCUPATION

By keeping occupation at the center of instructional design, the SCIL-OT Model naturally encourages that assessment targets students' understandings of occupation and health.

Occupation analysis is a foundational skill in occupational therapy education and is commonly used as an assignment across programs. How such assignments are constructed, however, matters with regard to what learning is actually assessed. Educators should consider which aspects of occupation are explicitly assessed in both the assignment instructions and the grading criteria.

Let's compare two examples as represented in Tables 5.7 and 5.8.

Table 5.7 Excerpts from the instructions for an activity analysis assessment illustrating unclear expectations related to students' understanding of occupation.

Instructions for an activity analysis assessment	
Select one of the following activities of daily living to analyze: • Walking the dog • Riding a bicycle along the river • Washing dinner dishes • Using an automatic teller machine to withdraw cash	◄ Includes specific occupations but lacks context: - No rationale as to why these were chosen; e.g., are they particularly relevant to the local context of the occupational therapy program? - The instructor could have chosen, for example, particular occupations known to be prominent or problematic in the local setting. E.g., going to a movie with friends at a cinema in a rural/remote area might be known to be difficult due to physical distance to a cinema and poor public transport.
Complete the occupation yourself and analyze the occupation and write about the following; a. Briefly describe the occupation. b. Describe the tools, materials, and equipment used. c. Describe the physical environment. d. Describe the social and cultural demands. e. List the sequential steps (no more than 15) of the occupation. f. Using any published list of skills (e.g., Occupational Therapy Practice Framework), identify 5–10 skills critical to this occupation. g. Briefly list the body structures and functions used during the occupation. h. List potential safety hazards.	◄ Includes all the standard sections of occupation analysis: - The verbs that preface each item indicate relatively low-level engagement with the process—describe, list, identify. - There is some consideration of limited aspects of the dynamics of occupation; i.e., there are some person factors and environment factors, but students only need to name or identify, and therefore there is no requirement for students to consider the transactions and the multidirectional relationships between the factors. - Importantly, there is no requirement for students to link occupational performance and engagement with health and well-being.

Table 5.8 Excerpts from the instructions for an activity analysis assessment illustrating clearer expectations related to students' understanding of occupation.

Instructions for an activity analysis assessment	
Why is this assessment important? It is well recognized that occupation, although seemingly mundane and every day, is a complex and multifaceted phenomenon. In order to work effectively as an occupational therapist, you must develop high-level knowledge and skills in occupation analysis. You will continue to develop expertise in occupation analysis throughout your undergraduate program, but this assessment will enable you to demonstrate your beginning knowledge and abilities.	◄ Highlighting the inherent complexity of occupation. ◄ The "why" of the assessment is linked to the "why" of the profession.
Through completion of this assessment, you need to demonstrate your value of an occupational perspective of humans, health and well-being, as well as individual and cultural differences.	◄ Captures dynamics of occupation—link between views of humans, occupation and health, culture.
For this assessment, you are required to write a 1,500-word report that analyzes a single recent instance of an occupation in which you have personally engaged. You can choose any occupation but it must be something that is a regular part of your life and not something that you have only performed once.	◄ A single, recent instance of a specific occupation.
You need to complete an analysis of a single recent instance of the occupation and describe how it impacted on your health and well-being.	◄ The task is to both analyze the specific occupation and consider its impact on health (dynamics of occupation).
Your occupation analysis must use the Canadian Model of Occupational Performance and Engagement (CMOP-E; Polatajko et al., 2013) as the guiding framework.	◄ Use of a specific and recognized occupation-centered framework to support students in analyzing, categorizing the specific occupation and the

The latter example of assessment instructions guides students to develop high-level reasoning within a clear occupational perspective. It also reinforces the SCIL-OT Model's emphasis on integrating occupation with context, personal experience, and health.

CURRICULUM DESIGN ACTIVITY: EVALUATING AND STRENGTHENING CONNECTIONS BETWEEN SPECIFIC OCCUPATIONS AND THE DYNAMICS OF OCCUPATION

The following exercise may be completed individually or collaboratively with other members of the faculty group. It supports ongoing refinement of teaching practices aligned with the SCIL-OT Model's emphasis on integrative, subject-centered learning.

The lines represent a continuum from Weak to Strong.

- **At the Weak end:** Documents and materials do not explicitly and consistently explain how specific occupations relate to the dynamics of occupations. Or students are not explicitly and consistently required to connect specific occupations to the dynamics linking occupation to health and well-being.
- **At the Strong end:** Documents and materials clearly and robustly feature the dynamics of occupation. Or students are explicitly and consistently required to connect specific occupations to the dynamics linking occupation to health and well-being.
- **In the middle:** Connections between occupation and health and well-being are present but could be more explicit or may not be integrated into how students are assessed.

Instructions

- Rate the strength of connection-making at each level of your program or teaching by marking an X on the continuum between Weak and Strong.
- Then, identify three ways connections between specific occupations and health and well-being could be strengthened at each level.

Note: Suggestions for strengthening may be minor but impactful. For example:

- Add a question to class preparation materials asking students to specifically relate the session's topics to specific occupations and to their relationship to health and well-being, or

- Add an instruction to an assignment.
- Revise rubrics to assess students' ability to connect specific occupations to their relationship to health.

Small changes like these can have a substantial impact.

Connections from Specific Occupation to Dynamics of Occupation in Key Curriculum Documents (Vision, Mission, Philosophy)

Weak ———————————————— Strong

Three suggestions to strengthen connections at the program level:

1.
2.
3.

Course Materials and Assignments Emphasize Connections between Specific Occupations and Dynamics of Occupation

Weak ———————————————— Strong

Three suggestions to strengthen connections at the course level:

1.
2.
3.

Class Session Processes Emphasize Making Connections between Specific Occupations and Dynamics of Occupation

Weak ———————————————— Strong

Three suggestions to strengthen connections at the class session level:

1.
2.
3.

Practice Education Emphasizes Connections between Specific Occupations and Dynamics of Occupation

Weak ———————————————— Strong

Three suggestions to strengthen connections at the practice education level:

1.
2.
3.

CONCLUSION

Occupation is at the center of the SCIL-OT Model. It is placed centrally in the model because it is the big idea of occupational therapy that which must be central to all practice and therefore entry-level education. Using the SCIL-OT reminds educators that all decisions about programs, courses, classroom activities, assessments, and practice education must be taken with consideration of how they contribute to students' knowledge, skills, and attitudes concerning occupation, and the relationship between occupation and health and well-being. However, it is insufficient to merely place occupation at the center. As indicated in the model, and elaborated in the chapters that follow, the links between occupation, topics, and the knowledge community must be deliberately created through learning activities and learning assessment to ensure a truly integrated and transformational educational experience for students.

REFERENCES

Canty, G., Roberts, M., & Molineux, M. (2020). Characteristics of occupation-based education within entry-level occupational therapy programs. *Journal of Occupational Therapy Education, 4*(2). https://encompass.eku.edu/jote/vol4/iss2/2

Chapparo, C., Ranka, J., & Nott, M. (2017). Occupational performance model (Australia): A description of constructs, structure and propositions. In M. Curtin, M. Egan, & J. Adams (Eds.), *Occupational therapy for people experiencing illness, injury or impairment: Promoting occupation and participation* (7th ed., pp. 134–147). Elsevier.

Craik, J., Davis, J., & Polatajko, H. (2013). Introducing the Canadian Practice Process Framework (CPPF): Amplifying the context. In E. Townsend & H. Polatajko (Eds.), *Enabling occupation II: Advancing an occupational therapy vision for health, well-being, & justice through occupation* (2nd ed., pp. 229–245). Canadian Association of Occupational Therapists.

Davis, J., Craik, J., & Polatajko, H. (2013). Using the Canadian Practice Process Framework (CPPF): Amplifying the process. In E. Townsend & H. Polatajko (Eds.), *Enabling occupation II: Advancing an occupational therapy vision for health, well-being, & justice through occupation* (2nd ed., pp. 247–272). Canadian Association of Occupational Therapists.

Hansen, E. (2011). *Idea-based learning: A course design process to promote conceptual understanding*. Stylus Publishing.

Humphry, R., & Wakeford, L. (2005). An occupation-centered discussion of development and implications for practice. *American Journal of Occupational Therapy, 50*(3), 258–257.

Kielhofner, G. (2009). *Conceptual foundations of occupational therapy practice* (4th ed.). F. A. Davis.

Molineux, M. (2009). The nature of occupation. In M. Curtin, M. Molineux, & J. Supyk-Mellson (Eds.), *Occupational therapy and physical dysfunction: Enabling occupation* (6th ed., pp. 17–25). Elsevier.

Polatajko, H., Davis, J., Stewart, D., Cantin, N., Amoroso, B., Purdie, L., & Zimmerman, D. (2013). Specifying the domain of concern: Occupation as core. In E. Townsend & H. Polatajko (Eds.), *Enabling occupation II: Advancing an occupational therapy vision for health, well-being, & justice through occupation* (2nd ed., pp. 13–35). Canadian Association of Occupational Therapists.

World Federation of Occupational Therapists. (2012). Definitions of occupational therapy from member organisations. World Federation of Occupational Therapists. https://www.wfot.org/resources/definitions-of-occupational-therapy-from-member-organisations

World Federation of Occupational Therapists. (2016). *Minimum standards for the education of occupational therapists*. Author.

Yerxa, E. (1998). Occupation: The keystone of a curriculum for a self-defined profession. *American Journal of Occupational Therapy, 52*(5), 355–372.

Chapter 6

Connecting Topics to Occupation

INTRODUCTION

As introduced in Chapter 4, each element in the SCIL-OT Model is connected by lines—these lines represent the essential work educators do to help students make meaningful connections across the curriculum. The topics learned in a curriculum are important, but only if they are learned in relation to the core of the profession, which is occupation. For a student to understand and apply a topic apart from the core is a learning achievement; however, it does not help the student develop their unique professional identity or fulfill their societal responsibility, as discussed in Chapter 1.

This chapter, therefore, focuses on the connections that educators must help students make between topics, represented by the stars in Figure 6.1, and the core of occupation.

Without making these connections in deliberate and explicit ways, educators run the risk that students perceive topics as stand-alone, disconnected from the core of occupation, and perceive occupation as simply another topic among topics rather than the central organizing dynamic of their professional knowledge.

Helping students make these connections clarifies why topics matter. Topics either help us understand the core of our profession more deeply or enhance the power of occupation as a therapeutic tool—both of which are essential for effective occupational therapy practice.

DOI: 10.4324/9781003635628-8

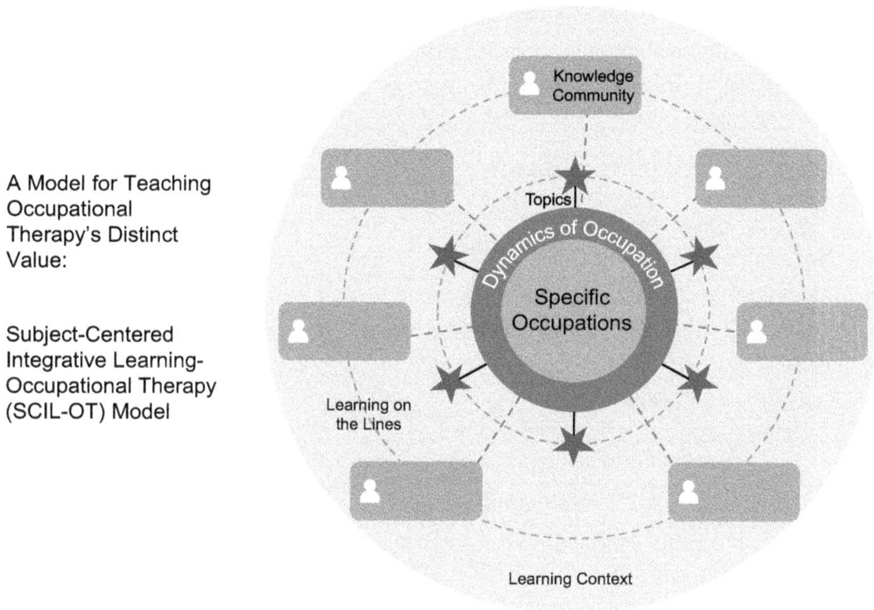

Figure 6.1 Educators design and assess learning on-the-line between topics (stars) and occupation.

OBJECTIVES

This chapter will help educators to:

1. Design learning opportunities that help students connect topics to the core subject of occupation.
2. Incorporate the connections between topics and core across the four component areas of a curriculum: the education program, the courses, the classroom, and practice education.
3. Assess and strengthen the topics to core connection across the four component areas of a curriculum.

TOPIC-TO-CORE CONNECTIONS

As conceptualized in the SCIL-OT Model, the profession's core concept of occupation encompasses specific occupations and the dynamics of occupation (see Chapters 2 and 4). While the SCIL-OT Model clearly places significant emphasis on the core of occupation, it also recognizes that other types of knowledge are required to practice occupational therapy effectively.

Of particular interest in this chapter are what are referred to in the model as *topics*. Topics are the many and varied but discrete knowledge, skills, and attitudes that are required either to understand occupation as deeply as is required to master it as a therapeutic tool or to support the use of occupation in practice with clients. For example, topics might include the following

- Evidence-based practice
- Manual muscle testing
- Motivational interviewing
- Knowledge of social structures and organizations
- Anatomy
- Theories of development
- Building codes and standards
- Schizophrenia
- Treatment options for rheumatoid arthritis

The list is actually endless.

Each program and educator, therefore, makes determinations about which topics will and will not be part of the program, course, or class session. Such decisions are often based on the program's intended outcomes, curricular history, the educators' expertise and preferences, the needs of affiliated practice sites, and other influential factors.

The task of educators is to create learning and assessment experiences so that students can make connections between the selected list of topics and the core of the profession. For example, learning and assessment strategies help students make connections such as the following:

- How does the *anatomy* of the knee joint contribute to our understanding of human occupation, and how does it help us design effective therapeutic experiences for clients?
- How do *building regulations* enable and/or inhibit human engagement in occupation?
- Why does the *welfare system* of a particular country selectively support some members of the community to engage in occupations that impact their health and well-being positively, but not all members of the community?
- How might the side effects of *antipsychotic drugs* impact a person's ability to wash and dress in the morning?

Based on how educators themselves understand such connections, they create learning outcomes, course descriptions, class activities, and learning assessments to emphasize the connections. While many occupational therapy programs might include content that addresses the parts of the preceding questions that pertain to topics (i.e., the first concept in each question), what is sometimes missing are explicit strategies that help students link the topics to occupation and occupational therapy (the second part of each question).

We know that we cannot merely assume or hope that students will make these links on their own; rather, we must intentionally design learning and assessment experiences to help students make the connections and, in doing so, support their learning 'on-the-lines' between topics and the core of occupation

CONNECTING TOPICS-TO-CORE AT THE PROGRAM LEVEL

One important task at the program level is, of course, deliberately and thoughtfully selecting which topics will be included in the program and which topics will be excluded, given that the potential list of topics is endless. Once this selection is made, the next task is to consider how connections between selected topics and the core of occupation can be made explicit in program-level documents. The following illustrations and curriculum design activities can support topic-to-core connections at the program level, including within learning outcomes (Boxes 6.1 and 6.2) and the program philosophy (Boxes 6.3 and 6.4).

While some might argue that topics—because they are not at the core of the profession—should not be elevated to the level of program aims, philosophy, and learning outcomes, this view likely underestimates the importance of continually linking topics to the core.

BOX 6.1 TWO EXAMPLES TO ILLUSTRATE CREATING CLEAR TOPICS-TO-CORE CONNECTIONS IN PROGRAM LEARNING OUTCOMES

One program might include a learning outcome that states

> *"By the end of the curriculum, students will apply in-depth knowledge of contemporary theories and approaches in the biomedical and health sciences."*

While this is a reasonable outcome, it does not make explicit the link between biomedical theories and occupation. Instead, it prioritizes topic knowledge, and by listing it as one of a few program-level outcomes, it may communicate a view of occupational therapy that prioritizes biomedical and health science perspectives. Further, as a program outcome, it mandates program evaluation focus on students' ability to apply biomedical and health sciences theories, a skill they may have acquired in the program, but does that skill as stated capture what the program most desires for student outcomes?

Consider an alternative program-level learning outcome:

> *"Students will demonstrate understanding of the determinants of occupation, including anatomical, neurological, psychological, socio-cultural, and environmental determinants."*

This outcome honors a range of topics (e.g., anatomy, psychology) and explicitly links them to occupation. More than that, it reframes the topics to show why they matter: these topics are important because they co-determine whether someone can engage in occupation, how easily they do so, or how difficult it may be.

The following curriculum design activity guides an assessment of your program's learning outcomes.

BOX 6.2 CURRICULUM DESIGN ACTIVITY TO EVALUATE PROGRAM LEARNING OUTCOMES

Review the learning outcomes for your program. Indicate which, if any, outcomes emphasize topics without their connections to occupation. Rewrite the objective to emphasize learning the topics in relation to occupation.

BOX 6.3 TWO SAMPLES FROM PROGRAMS' PHILOSOPHY STATEMENTS, ILLUSTRATING CLARIFYING AND DEEPENING TOPICS-TO-CORE CONNECTIONS IN THESE STATEMENTS

One program philosophy includes this sentence:

> *"Participation in those meaningful occupations impacts health at all levels including physical, psychosocial, and spiritual health."*

This statement signals that engagement in occupation impacts physical, psychosocial, and spiritual health—all of which are topics. Yet in this sentence, they are clearly linked to occupation.

This statement could be strengthened by recognizing the two-way relationship between those topics and occupation. As currently written, it does not acknowledge how different physical, psychosocial, and spiritual health statuses can influence a person's ability to engage in occupation.

Consider an alternative statement:

> *"People's participation in their occupations impacts, positively and not so positively, all levels of health—including physical, psychosocial, and spiritual health. Simultaneously, people's health statuses (physical, psychosocial, and spiritual) influence their participation in occupation."*

This version makes the reciprocal relationship explicit, helping students and educators see how topics and core are interdependent.

Consider your own program philosophy using the following design activity.

BOX 6.4 CURRICULUM DESIGN ACTIVITY: PROGRAM PHILOSOPHY

GUIDELINES

- Review your program philosophy.
- Circle statements that emphasize topics in relation to occupation.
- Underline statements that omit or only implicitly refer to the connection.
- Rephrase the underlined statements to emphasize the importance of the topics in relation to occupation.

CONNECTING TOPICS-TO-CORE AT THE COURSE LEVEL

Building a curriculum with integrated topics is challenging. It often results in courses being named according to topics, which can create pressure to teach those topics, and create student expectations to learn those topics, in a stand-alone fashion. For example, course might be called Ergonomics, Neuroscience and Neurodevelopment, Upper Limb Orthoses and Rehabilitation, Pathophysiology, Kinesiology, Musculoskeletal Anatomy, or Assistive Technology.

While there are valid reasons for including these courses in an occupational therapy program, their names do not clearly communicate to students how the content relates to the central idea of the profession—occupation. Some may view this as a minor concern, but students often interpret course titles as indicators of importance, thinking:

> *"If we have a whole course on neuroscience, that topic must be important in itself." They may even think that neuroscience must be foundational knowledge for occupational therapy.*

When possible, the naming should signal the relationship between the topic and the core of the profession. Consider the following illustration (Box 6.5).

BOX 6.5 ILLUSTRATION OF COURSE NAMING TO EMPHASIZE TOPICS-TO-CORE CONNECTIONS

The following titles link the topic with the core by explicitly naming or suggesting the relationship. Mental health conditions (topics) are important for occupational therapists because they affect a person's ability to perform and engage in occupations. Making such connections visible in course titles helps students see relationships that educators may take for granted.

- Impact of Mental Health on Occupational Performance and Experience
- Influences on Occupational Performance: Conditions and Interventions

At one level, naming a course after its primary topic can be easily addressed by renaming the course to reflect the connection between the primary topic or topics to occupation. At another level, simply modifying the course name is not sufficient if the design of the course does not reflect the link named in the title. That is, if other elements of the course—such as the objectives, description, and assessments—do not also link topics to occupation.

Course learning outcomes are a key opportunity to explicitly document the topics-to-core connections. Driven by the outcomes, the course assessments will then naturally assess students' ability to make the connections.

In a course focused on enabling occupation for people with mental health conditions, the outcomes in Box 6.6 make the link clear for students and help them stay alert to those connections.

BOX 6.6 SAMPLE COURSE LEARNING OUTCOMES WRITTEN TO FOCUS LEARNING ON THE TOPICS-TO-CORE CONNECTIONS

- Describe the impact of mental health and mental illness on occupational performance and participation.
- Apply theoretical frameworks when reasoning about occupational therapy interventions for people with mental health and mental illness.
- Plan appropriate occupational therapy interventions to enhance the occupational performance and participation of people with mental health problems and mental illness.
- Demonstrate consideration of context when planning occupational therapy interventions, including personal, practice, cultural, legislative, and ethical contexts.

TIP: *Write outcomes using language that teaches students the focus of occupational therapy interventions is the enhancement of occupational performance.*

TIP: *Since outcomes guide learning assessments, keeping the outcome targeted on the link between a topic and occupation will lead to assessing learning at the link.*

Course descriptions are another opportunity to make the link between topics and the core explicit for students. Once clear objectives are established, course descriptions can be crafted to reinforce the same connections to occupation that are captured in the objectives (Box 6.7).

BOX 6.7 ILLUSTRATING HOW COURSE DESCRIPTIONS MAY CONVEY TOPICS IN ISOLATION FROM OCCUPATION, SHIFTING THE FOCUS OF LEARNING AND ASSESSMENT TOWARD DISCREET SKILLS AND AWAY FROM HOW THE SKILLS SERVE OCCUPATIONAL PERFORMANCE, ENGAGEMENT, AND EXPERIENCE

Consider the following course description for a course titled, *Therapeutic Skills I: Biomechanics.* Note that the description lacks clear topic-to-core connections:

> *The purpose of this course is to provide the student with lecture and laboratory study that will focus on using the Biomechanical Frame of Reference for assessment and intervention. Students gain skills in analysis of movement, muscle palpation, goniometry of range of motion, and manual muscle testing. Students will acquire knowledge and skills in administering standardized hand strength tests, and assessments for edema. Adjunct treatment utilizing superficial thermal modalities will be introduced, with assessment of blood pressure, and pulse rate for patient care. Of primary concern will be integration of assessment skills and application to biomechanical intervention approaches, and intensive opportunity and practice in professional and peer communication skills.*

This description emphasizes discrete skills within the biomechanical frame of reference but does not explain how those skills relate to occupational performance, engagement, or experience.

In contrast, the following course description (Table 6.1) refers to the topic-to-core link, albeit briefly:

Table 6.1 Illustrating course description with a weak mention of the topics-to-core connection.

Course title and description	
Foundations of Occupation: Neuroscience—Application of basic neural function to the analysis of daily living tasks and activities; review of pathological conditions that interfere with performance in occupation.	◄ The topic of basic neural function is linked to analysis of daily living tasks and activities. ◄ Topic of pathological conditions linked to occupation as one factor that may disrupt performance.

TIP: *Further strengthen by using the term occupation or occupational performance and engagement for daily living tasks. Consider conveying a bi-directional relationship between neural development/function and occupational engagement, for example, how occupation impacts pathological conditions.*

The course description in Table 6.2 makes the topics-to-core connections explicit.

Table 6.2 Illustrating how course descriptions can be used to explicitly reinforce the topics-to-core connections.

Course title and description	
. . . explores the structures, functions, and processes of the human body that support participation in occupation. The course will focus on neurological systems, mental processes, sensory processing, digestion, reproduction, endocrine, and immune responses that support human occupation.	◄ Topics presented as supporting participation in occupation

TOPICS-TO-CORE CONNECTIONS AT THE CLASS SESSION LEVEL

Classroom learning activities need to make clear that topics are topics; that is, they are not unique or defining aspects of occupational therapy knowledge and skill. They are, however, important and valuable for how they illuminate aspects of occupation or contribute to how people engage in and experience occupation.

This can be achieved by helping students understand that the knowledge required to practice occupational therapy comprises different types of knowledge and by providing opportunities for students to step back and examine the structure of professional knowledge.

For example, Kielhofner (2009) proposed that professional knowledge includes three types:

- *Paradigm knowledge:* defines "the nature and purpose of the field" and describes the "cultural core" of the profession. It is unique and defining of occupational therapy.
- *Related knowledge:* includes knowledge and skills that are not unique to occupational therapy but are useful and often specific to a practice context. This is akin to topics in the SCIL-OT.

- *Conceptual practice models:* provide guidance on how to integrate and apply paradigm and related knowledge in practice.

These categories remind educators that related knowledge and conceptual models must be represented in direct relation to the core. Box 6.8 offers an example of an in-class learning activity to help students understand the layers of professional knowledge.

Once students understand this structure, they can be guided through a critical reflection and discussion about where specific pieces of knowledge are located and how they relate to each other.

BOX 6.8 ILLUSTRATION OF AN IN-CLASS ACTIVITY TO TEACH TYPES OF KNOWLEDGE, HELPING STUDENTS UNDERSTAND HOW TOPICS RELATE TO THE CORE PARADIGM OF THE PROFESSION

To do this, the educator presents students with examples of occupational therapy knowledge and asks them to categorize each as *paradigm*, *conceptual practice model*, or *related knowledge*, using only the information provided.

Students receive two to three cards, each with one item. The cards could be numerous; for example, each of these topics could be a card:

- Client-centered practice
- Knowledge of human anatomy
- Assessment of cooking
- Using a goniometer
- Ability to modify any occupation to improve clients' occupational engagement
- Understanding of the relationship between occupation and health and well-being
- Stress management techniques
- Use of cooking to improve upper limb weakness
- Knowledge of legislation impacting on people with mental health conditions
- Motivational interviewing

Students then place their cards under the appropriate category and explain their reasoning. These explanations are then used to

- clarify the distinctions between types of knowledge.

- help students identify what is a topic and what is core.
- show how a topic becomes useful when linked to the core.

For example, students may initially argue that client-centered practice is core. But when prompted to consider its origins in psychology and its use across professions, they realize it is not unique to occupational therapy. This opens a discussion:

- Client-centered practice is valuable in occupational therapy only when it helps us understand the client as an occupational being.
- Used in isolation, it lacks relevance; connected to occupation, it enhances practice.

This activity helps students see that topics are subordinate—but not irrelevant—to the core of occupation.

Discussions such as this can of course be stimulated in classes in many different ways. The key for all of them, however, is to not dismiss topics as irrelevant because they are in themselves not occupational. Instead, it is to help students understand that topics are helpful in occupational therapy when they are connected to the core, hence the connecting lines in the SCIL-OT and the principle that learning occurs on-the-lines. Framing topics in this way helps students locate topic knowledge as subordinate, but not irrelevant, to the core of occupation.

TOPICS-TO-CORE CONNECTIONS IN PRACTICE EDUCATION

Practice education is a crucial aspect of all occupational therapy programs and offers a key opportunity for students to learn and apply topic knowledge in real-world settings. However, students can often feel overwhelmed by the number of topics required to practice in a particular setting.

For example, working in a service that provides occupational therapy for people following hand injuries requires knowledge and skills related to

- hand anatomy, kinesiology, and physiology (often in greater depth than other settings).
- common hand injuries and conditions.
- wound healing.
- splints and orthoses.
- psychological impact of trauma.

- medical and surgical terminology.
- hand and upper limb assessment tools and techniques.

While this example reflects a highly specialized practice area, educators should remember that many practice areas may feel equally complex and specialized to students, even if experienced therapists consider them routine. Box 6.9 provides an example of how practice educators can support students in making topic-to-core connections.

BOX 6.9 INSTRUCTIONAL DESIGN ACTIVITY SUPPORTING TOPICS-TO-CORE CONNECTIONS IN PRACTICE EDUCATION

Practice educators can support students in making topic-to-core connections using exercises like the following:

- Require students to create a list of topics that are vital to understand in their practice setting. If the list is long, sequence the topics—identify which are most important early in the placement and which can be addressed later as the student's confidence grows.
- Beside each topic or category, have students describe its link to the core of occupation. For example:
  - A particular assessment tool might evaluate a client's performance and engagement in occupations such as writing or cooking.
  - Understanding the psychological impact of trauma can help students grasp the dynamics of occupation—such as how a client feels about returning to work after an injury.
- Give students continuous opportunities to make these links, through:
  - Questioning: "How does this assessment relate to this person's occupations?"
  - Explanation: "I chose this assessment because it informs me of potential barriers to the client's priority occupation of eating without assistance."
- Require students to make these links explicitly in the following:
  - Client discussions
  - Interprofessional communication
  - Documentation
  - Written reflections and other learning activities

Using the SCIL-OT Model in practice education reminds educators to teach 'on-the-lines'—so that students not only learn the topics relevant to their setting but also understand how those topics relate to the core of occupation. Practice educators already do an excellent job of teaching the nuances of their settings; the SCIL-OT Model encourages them to anchor those topics to occupation. One possible process includes considering the following questions with students:

1. What are the topics that are important in this practice area or setting?
2. How do those topics link to specific occupations typically addressed with clients in this setting?
3. How do those topics link to the dynamics of occupation in support of optimizing client health and well-being.
4. How might students' abilities to make those links be scaffolded across the placement and client journeys?
5. What opportunities exist in the placement for the student to explain the topics-to-core connections to others (clients, team members, payors, etc.)?

ASSESSING STUDENTS KNOWLEDGE, SKILLS, AND APTITUDE AT THE TOPIC-TO-CORE CONNECTION

Because assessment is often seen as determining whether students know or can apply specific material, it can seem relatively straightforward. Consider these two questions from a written examination:

- Short answer question: Describe, giving examples, the characteristics of a typical synovial joint.
- Multiple choice question: Which carpal bone articulates with the radius?
    - Trapezoid
    - Scaphoid
    - Hamate
    - Pisiform
    - Capitate

These are excellent questions for assessing related knowledge of human anatomy—an important topic—but they would be equally appropriate for any health professional. There is no linking to the core of occupation. Students could score well on an exam filled with these types of questions and still lack understanding of how that knowledge is relevant to specific occupations or the dynamics of occupation. It is important to design assess students' knowledge at the connection of the topics we teach and the core.

Alternative questions that assess topics-to-core knowledge are illustrated in Table 6.3.

Table 6.3 Examples of exam questions illustrating assessment of students' knowledge at the topics-to-core connection.

Exam prompts	
Short answer question: Jordan *works as a wood furniture maker* and has recently sustained an injury to the thumb on his dominant hand. Explain how the carpometacarpal joint of the thumb, on Jordan's dominant hand, would have contributed to holding a hammer prior to his injury.	◀ The prompt foregrounds a specific occupation and asks students to demonstrate their anatomical knowledge in direct connection to a specific occupation.
Multiple choice question: Which of the following muscles is least likely to be used *when a person grips a steering wheel while driving a car?* a) Flexor digitorum profundus b) Flexor digitorum superficialis c) Abductor pollicis brevis d) Lumbricales	◀ Anatomical knowledge is assessed in direct relation to the specific occupation of driving. ◀ This prompt could be strengthened with more detail and by placing occupation first, e.g., when a person grips a steering wheel while driving a car, placing two hands around the wheel at the positions of 10 and 12 o'clock (imaging the circle of the steering wheel as a clock), which of the following muscles are least likely to be used?

These questions are only slightly different from the originals. The anatomical knowledge is still tested, but the questions guide students to explicitly link the topic to occupation and support educators in assessing their ability to do so. The questions signal to students, "You need to know this topic in relation to how it enables or inhibits occupational performance and engagement." Assessments that require students to connect topics-to-core simultaneously help them embody the professional reasoning of occupational therapists.

The same principle used for exams above can be also applied to written assignments and to presentations. For example, a written assessment might ask students to interpret a range of evaluation results—such as range of motion, memory scores, cognitive assessments, interview notes, and a home assessment report—and write an intervention plan with full justification for selected interventions.

To ensure students make topic-to-core connections, the assignment could ask them to

- identify an occupational challenge for the client.
- select only those assessment findings that may contribute to that challenge.
- explain their reasoning, linking person or environment factors directly to the specific occupation/s in the case.

This approach requires students to connect assessment data to the dynamics of occupation, reinforcing the SCIL-OT principle that learning happens 'on-the-lines.'

CURRICULUM DESIGN ACTIVITY: EVALUATING AND STRENGTHENING TOPIC-TO-CORE CONNECTION MAKING

The following exercise may be completed individually or collaboratively with other members of the faculty group. It supports ongoing refinement of teaching practices aligned with the SCIL-OT Model's emphasis on integrative, subject-centered learning.

The lines represent a continuum from Weak to Strong.

- **At the Weak end:** Program documents do not explicitly and consistently link topics to specific occupations or the dynamics of occupations OR Students are not explicitly and consistently required to connect topics to specific occupations or to the dynamics linking occupation to health and well-being.
- **At the Strong end:** Program documents clearly and robustly link topics to occupation OR Students are explicitly and consistently required to connect topics to specific occupations or to the dynamics linking occupation to health and well-being.
- **In the middle:** Topic-to-core connections are present but may remain part of the instructors' background rationale in course designs or may not be integrated into how students are assessed.

Instructions:

- Rate the strength of topic-to-core connection-making at each level of your program or teaching by marking an X on the continuum between Weak and Strong.
- Then, identify three ways topic-to-core connection-making could be strengthened at each level.

Note: Suggestions for strengthening may be minor but impactful. For example:

- Add a question to class preparation materials asking students to specifically relate the session's topics to specific occupations and to their relationship to health and well-being, or
- Add an instruction to an assignment.
- Revise rubrics to assess students' ability to connect topics to the core of occupation.

Small changes like these can have a substantial impact.

Topics-to-Core Connections in Key Curriculum Documents (Vision, Mission, Philosophy)

Weak ———————————————— Strong

Three suggestions to strengthen connections at the program level:

1.
2.
3.

Course Materials and Assignments Emphasize Topic-to-Core Connections

Weak ———————————————— Strong

Three suggestions to strengthen connections at the course level:

1.
2.
3.

Class Session Processes Emphasize Making Topic-to-Core Connections

Weak ——————————————— Strong

Three suggestions to strengthen connections at the class session level:

1.
2.
3.

Practice Education Emphasizes Topic-to-Core Connections

Weak ——————————————— Strong

Three suggestions to strengthen connections during practice education:

1.
2.
3.

CONCLUSION

This chapter has focused on making explicit the link between the many different topics covered in occupational therapy curricula and the core subject of occupation. While educators may already see these connections, it is essential to design learning activities and learning assessments that support students in seeing them too and to make those links clear and unmistakable for themselves.

By doing so, educators help students make sense of what might otherwise feel like a never-ending list of disconnected content areas. When students learn topics in relationship to the core of occupation, they not only understand why those topics are important but also reinforce the centrality and primacy of occupation in their professional identity and reasoning.

REFERENCES

Kielhofner, G. (2009). *Conceptual foundations of occupational therapy practice* (4th ed.). F. A. Davis.

Chapter 7

Connecting Topics to Other Topics

INTRODUCTION

Chapter 7 examines how educators help students learn to connect the enormous array of topics they are expected to grasp and master throughout their education. As described in Chapter 4, topics in the SCIL-OT Model refer to what we, as educators, explain, demonstrate, and include in instructional materials.

Among countless possibilities, topics encompass what students must understand conceptually, for example, human development across the lifespan, occupational justice, or various theories and conceptual practice models.

Topics also include numerous skills that are inextricably linked to conceptual understanding—such as analyzing and adapting everyday occupations and environments, conducting occupational profiles, or assessing the needs of community agencies. Indeed, the topics students encounter over the course of their education can appear endless and overwhelming.

As discussed in Chapter 3, the SCIL-OT Model is heavily influenced by the theoretical framework of *integrative learning*. Integrative learning is especially relevant to the focus of this chapter; namely, designing learning to ensure that students explicitly link interrelated topics to one another and to the core subject of occupation. Integrative learning occurs when students connect topics that are relevant to particular situations within an occupational perspective, and thereby learn processes for addressing complex and evolving societal concerns. Conversely, integrative learning is obstructed when students solely learn isolated topics or are solely assessed on their knowledge of isolated topics.

The purpose of Chapter 7 is to illustrate and examine ways to strengthen topic-to-topic connection-making within an occupational perspective. This examination

DOI: 10.4324/9781003635628-9

occurs across the four components of a curriculum introduced in Chapter 1: (1) the education program, (2) courses, (3) class sessions, and (4) practice education.

OBJECTIVES

This chapter will help educators to:

1. Design learning opportunities that help students connect diverse topics within an occupational perspective.
2. Identify and differentiate what constitutes topics across the four component areas of a curriculum: the education program, the courses, the classroom, and practice education.
3. Assess and strengthen topic-to-topic connection-making across the four component areas of a curriculum.

TOPIC-TO-TOPIC CONNECTIONS AT THE PROGRAM LEVEL

Examining and selecting topics from the *30,000-foot view* of an education program can feel overwhelming. This sense of overwhelm can lead us, as educators, to *default to accreditation standards* to determine which topics we ought to include in our curriculum, and which we can afford to leave out. We may also be tempted to default to traditional or conventional course structures in occupational therapy.

Yet rather than relying on accreditation standards or previously established courses, it is essential that we first identify the content and experiences that best express the top-tier elements of our program's curriculum design (AOTA, 2021). These top-tier elements often include a program's vision, mission, aim, philosophy, context, assessment plan, and overall outcomes. Each of these should:

- Clearly address occupation
- Reflect the features of the program's learning context
- Convey a contemporary or future-oriented view of occupational therapy

In addition, these elements should be congruent. That is:

- The *vision* should reflect the context and logically lead to the *mission or aim*
- The *mission/aim* should reflect the context and lead to the *outcomes*
- The *outcomes* should reflect the context and lead to the *assessment plan*
- All elements should be captured in—and brought to life by—the *program philosophy*

When inductively distilled from these top-tier curricular elements, topics at the program level take the form of larger unified wholes, or gestalts, that distinguish particular programs and reflect their highest aspirations and commitments.

To identify such gestalts, it helps to distinguish *large-content topics* from the *small-content topics* they encompass. A large-content topic is a meta-theme or knowledge area that is expressed across the key curriculum design documents, even implicitly. Large-content topics or themes are knowledge areas that without a focused emphasis, the program could not realize its vision and mission or achieve its outcomes or enliven its philosophy. For example:

- A program with a vision to enable the participation of individuals and communities in healthful occupations might distill occupation-focused assessments as one *large-content topic*.
  - Related *small-content topics* may be obtaining occupational profiles of individuals and communities, conducting occupational performance observations, locating epidemiologic data.
- Another *large-content topic* might be *enabling occupation skills*.
  - Related *small-content topics*: advocacy, coaching, educating.

Of course, there are ever-tinier topics within occupational profiles, observations, advocacy, and coaching. But for the purposes of identifying topics at the program level, and keeping them aligned with the curriculum design, it is important to avoid diving too deep into the smallest components. Instead, the aim is to identify larger themes and smaller topics that activate the curriculum design elements in support of students' integrative learning.

Figure 7.1 outlines a process of distilling themes and topics from the top-tier curricular elements (vision, mission, aim, philosophy, among others). Each of these holds implications for the large-content topics or themes the curriculum must include. The large-content topics may become curricular threads. In turn, each large-content topic, carefully defined, holds implications for the program's outcomes. The outcomes in turn determine the necessary small-content topics deemed essential for achieving the outcomes.

> **TIP:** *Only start identifying topics after establishing key curricular elements and program outcomes.*

Once topics associated with program outcomes are identified, we can then begin to discern patterns among these large themes and small topics and group them logically into "piles." These piles may become courses.

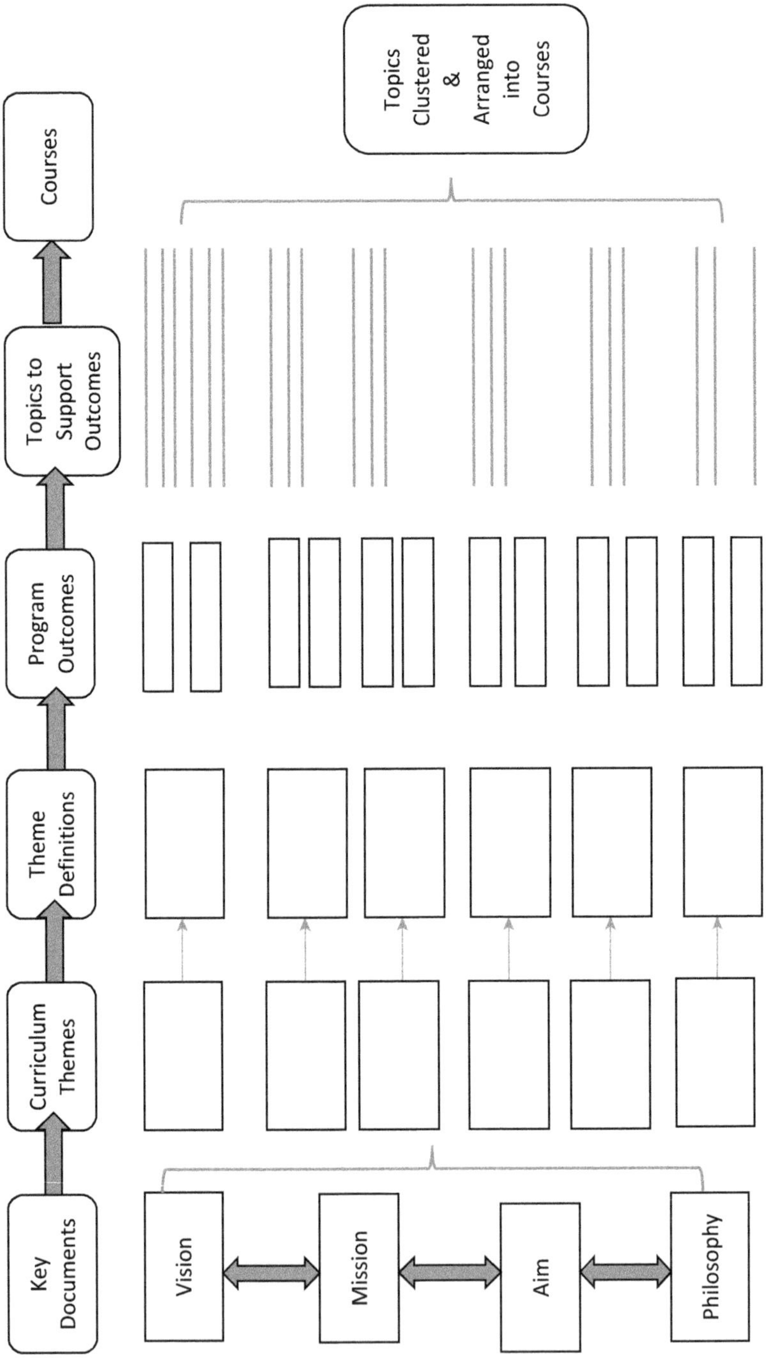

Figure 7.1 After centering occupation in all key curriculum documents and ensuring coherence among them, use an inductive process to generate themes, outcomes, topics, and courses from the key documents.

By following this (Table 7.1) or similar processes, we help ensure that the courses we design or revise have been distilled from the key elements of our curriculum rather than solely from external mandates.

Table 7.1 Illustrating topic-to-topic connections at the program level refers to distilling large-content themes and small-content topics directly from the key curricular documents.

Key curriculum documents	Vision Mission Aim Philosophy Context Curricular threads Program outcomes Strategic and evaluation plans
Distilled large-content themes (one example)	Innovation and everyday leadership
Theme definition	Everyday leadership refers to the big and small ways occupational therapists innovate each day as change agents in systems and with clients. Through formal and informal leadership, occupational therapists collaboratively coach people to change, develop products and processes that support how people do things, and create services that respond to population, community, and individual needs—thereby improving lives and promoting the profession.
Program outcomes associated with the theme	Graduates: 1. Assume formal and informal leadership roles, identify, and develop leadership styles, values, passions, skills, and growth areas while appreciating those of others.
	2. Conduct proficient environmental scans and use findings to inform leadership and innovation in systems.
	3. Collaboratively develop, test, and implement new ideas, discoveries and solutions that are cost-effective and meet occupational needs of specific populations, communities, and individuals (e.g., programs, products, businesses, service expansions)

Table 7.1 (Continued)

Small-content topics to support the outcomes	Definitions of leadership, leadership styles, personal strengths and growth areas, needs assessments, collaboration with stakeholders, professional leadership opportunities, relationships between leadership and enabling occupation, client-centered practice as leadership, leadership vs. position or role as leader, occupational therapy process and leadership process, how systems work, how systems change, enabling occupation skills and leadership.

BOX 7.1 CURRICULUM DESIGN ACTIVITY TO IDENTIFY LARGE-CONTENT THEMES AND SMALL-CONTENT TOPICS FROM THE PROGRAM-LEVEL DOCUMENTS

Guidelines. This activity consists of eight steps. As you take these steps, try to set aside, or bracket, your previous experiences with how occupational therapy topics, skills, and courses go together. Try also to bracket accreditation requirements. This bracketing will keep you open to new ways in which topics may connect, and thereby, new ways in which courses can be formulated to better help students achieve your program's overall aims and learning outcomes.

Furthermore, avoid veering off into general topics that students might need to learn or that you personally prefer they learn. Instead, stay close to what students specifically need to learn if the program is to fulfill its vision and bring its philosophy to life each day in classrooms.

Step 1. Gather the program's key curriculum design elements:

- Features of the learning context
- Vision, mission, aim, philosophy
- Prompt: Are the key curricular documents congruent with each other? Is occupation centered?

Step 2. Review each element using these prompts:

- For the *program vision* to come alive in what students learn, they will need some knowledge of . . . [list large-content themes]

- For the *program mission and aim* to come alive in what students learn, they will need some knowledge of . . . [list large-content themes]
- For the *program philosophy* to come alive in what students learn, they will need some knowledge of . . . [list large-content themes]
- [if an established program] If students are to achieve the *program outcomes as* evidenced by the assessment plan, they will need some knowledge of . . . [list large-content topics]

Step 3. Identify the large-content themes that appear most frequently across the lists you've compiled from the documents. If your documents are congruent, and if you've stayed close to what students specifically need to learn in relation to the curriculum design elements, these large-content themes will clearly reflect your curriculum.

Step 4. Working with the most frequently occurring large-content themes, clearly define each one. Document how they relate to each other.

Step 5. Working from the definition, generate 3–4 program outcomes that if achieved graduates would be said to embody the large-content theme.

Step 6. For each program outcome, ask: If students are to achieve a portion of the outcome what 6–8 small-content topics must they learn and connect? Observe your list of small-content topics.

Step 7. Based on the logical connections you've created in the above steps:

- Ask: What large themes and small content topics seem to naturally "group together"?
- Develop a tentative name for each grouping based on how the topics logically go together. These groupings may form *tentative courses*.

Step 8. Critical step.

Ask: How will students know about the connections you've created and documented among large and small topics?

To make the connections visible to students, consider the following approaches:

- *Create orientation activities* that help students discover how the large topics of the curriculum relate to one another.
- *Start each new course* with activities that help students 'bridge' from the previous semester and follow the logic of the curriculum-level topics.

- *End each semester* by 'bridging' to the next, showing how current topics connect to upcoming ones.
- *Ask students to create a concept map* at the end of each course showing how the course relates to previous large-content topics in the curriculum.

TOPIC-TO-TOPIC CONNECTIONS AT THE COURSE LEVEL

Topics at the course level abound in the materials that educators develop for particular courses. As noted earlier, topics at this level are distilled from—and aligned with—the top-tier curricular elements of programs. However, it is primarily through *course materials* that we draw students' attention to the *primary topics* of any given course.

A course's key topics are evident in multiple formats. For instance, topics are often embedded throughout course syllabi, especially in the formal course description, learning objectives, and units or foci of study. Topics are frequently posted for each class session on class schedules or course websites. They are often the focus of required readings and study guides that help students identify, understand, and interconnect multiple topics as they prepare for class. Indeed, topics—and the integrative learning strategies that support connection-making—can be ubiquitous in course materials. For these reasons, it is often the case that a curriculum's key topics are most readily visible at the course level.

At the same time, we are not always intentional or explicit in how our courses will require students to interrelate multiple topics and to grasp why connection-making is essential. The many connections among topics that we readily see as educators can remain invisible to students. Therefore, it can be helpful to explicitly identify the main topics that populate our course materials and to embed integrative learning strategies—or linking strategies—within them.

Attending to these design choices can strengthen students' focused attention and engagement in active connection-making experiences. To illustrate, the next section presents three samples of course materials:

1. A course description
2. A course schedule
3. A case study assignment

Course Descriptions

Table 7.2 illustrates a course description used to introduce the syllabus for *Occupational Performance for Adults and Older Adults (OTD 751)*. The table annotates the full course description to highlight topic-to-topic connections in the description. The key topics that students are expected to master throughout this course are not only clearly identifiable but also conceptually substantive and numerous.

The educator who wrote this course description intentionally emphasized connection-making. The description immediately signals that the topics students will learn in OTD 751 are linked to those in a companion course, OTD 752. It also clarifies that students are not simply learning to perform stand-alone assessments and interventions. Rather, the description communicates that students will learn to relate assessments and interventions to different understandings of occupational functioning, as represented in two distinct practice models, the companion course, and their fieldwork experiences.

Table 7.2 Sample course description annotated to illustrate making explicit topic-to-topic connections.

Course description with topics highlighted	
Occupational Performance for Adults and Older Adults is a companion course to OT 752.	◀ Topics are connected across two courses.
Both courses utilize the Occupational Functioning Model (OFM) and the Occupational Therapy Intervention Process Model (OTIPM) as guiding structures for learning.	◀ Conceptual and process models are used to organize the units, providing a format to link topics to each other and to a larger whole.
By guiding structures, we mean that (a) course units correspond to and progress through the elements of the models, and (b) the daily class structure also mirrors both models by introducing topics in a top-down sequence.	◀ The sequence of class sessions are designed to reflect the models' top-down approaches.

Table 7.2 (Continued)

In this course, you acquire the foundations for, and demonstrate competence in, assessments and interventions as they relate to these levels of occupational functioning: abilities, skills, and developed capacities. However, you must continually relate abilities, skills, and developed capacities to the levels of occupational functioning addressed in OT 752: self-efficacy, life role participation, competence, satisfaction, activities, and habits.	➤ The topics of assessment and intervention are connected to levels of occupational functioning in the model, each a topic.
Also this semester, you complete a 40-hour Level I Fieldwork where: (1) foundations and competencies achieved in this course and OT 752 are applied in a practice setting; (2) current practice in a variety of settings is analyzed according to all levels of the OFM and OTIPM; (3) various intervention approaches from the OTIPM are observed, including consultation, education, therapeutic use of self, occupation-based activity, purposeful activity, and preparatory methods;	➤ Topics are connected to concurrent course and to fieldwork, and theories are connected to practice.
and (4) feedback on performance is provided by fieldwork educators. Experiences and knowledge gained on Level I FW are brought back, discussed, and taught to peers in the course.	➤ Practice education is connected back to course topics.

Class Schedules and Units of Study

Table 7.3 shows the class schedule for a course titled *Kinesiology of Occupation*. Like the course description in Table 7.2, the topics students are expected to learn across the four units of study are readily apparent. Indeed, the foci of the class sessions comprise the course's major topics.

To help students better see *topic-to-topic connections*, the educator used a linking strategy: grouping topics into cohesive units. Specifically, the educator created four distinct units, each designed to support students in making sense of the course content:

- Unit I signals that the topics in the first two weeks are *critical foundations* for understanding what follows.

- Unit II helps students grasp the broader idea to which topics relate and how to make sense of them.
- Unit III conveys the larger point that the topics, when taken together, are intended to make.
- Unit IV turns students' attention to the main focus of the course.

Collectively, the names of the four units convey how the central focus of the course relates to broader concepts in the field, such as analyzing occupation and analyzing environments, terminology of anatomy and terminology of doing. This structuring strategy not only clarifies the course's intellectual arc but also supports students in integrating knowledge across sessions—a key principle of subject-centered learning.

Table 7.3 Sample class schedule organized by units illustrating how to emphasize topic-to-topic connections and topic-to-core connections.

Unit I: Foundational concepts for understanding kinesiology in an occupational therapy context	
Class session	Focus of study
1	Ways of knowing in studying human movement
2	Occupational therapy perspectives on human movement and body structures
Unit II: There are different languages for describing human movement in occupational contexts	
3	Languages of movement: anatomical
4	Languages of movement: biomechanical and kinesiological
5	Languages of movement: the language of *doing* is occupational therapy's language
Unit III: Occupational analyses involves multiple levels and languages	
6	Introduction to analyzing occupation and activity
7	Analyzing environments as a drivers of movement
8	Analyzing occupations as drivers of movement
9	Analyzing body functions and structures as supports to movement
10	Occupation when the body doesn't move
Unit IV: Biomechanical analysis during occupational performance	
End of illustration. Course continues through Week 16	

To help students group and connect topics throughout a course's progression, educators can build on the linking strategy of using units in the class schedule. In our experience, students often become focused on completing readings or study guides for a specific class and lose sight of the larger context—specifically, how the week's topics fit into the unit topics as a whole.

> **TIP:** *It helps to continuously orient students to the unit presently under consideration. Reviewing the logic of course units and topics each week is an integrative learning strategy that supports topic-to-topic connection-making.*

To reinforce this orientation, educators can build upon the structure of study units in the syllabus by explicitly referencing the unit in study guides and class discussions. For example, class sessions may begin with orienting statements like:

- "Today, we will wrap up the unit on language. In this unit, you learned that therapists use multiple languages to describe human movement."
- "Today we begin a new unit. In the previous unit, we explored language; in this unit, we put the different ways of talking about movement in the context of top-down assessment."

These small but intentional cues help students track the intellectual progression of the course, making it easier to integrate new topics with prior topics.

Written Assignments

Course assignments often require students to link multiple topics—sometimes without realizing it. Take, for example, the commonplace assignment of conducting an occupational interview. Students are often given instructions similar to those in Table 7.4. At first glance, this may seem like a 'simple' task, but note how many distinct topics students must connect to complete it successfully.

Sometimes this assignment goes even further. Students may be asked to:

- *Set goals* for the interviewee based on the data they collect,
- *Select interventions* to address those goals, or
- *Co-construct an occupation-based wellness plan* with the interviewee.

The question becomes:

1. How well do students understand that they had to *actively connect multiple topics* to complete the assignment?
2. Can they identify the *specific topics* they actually connected?

TIP: *Just as written class schedules can be structured to highlight topic connections, written assignments can include prompts that make connection-making explicit. For example, related to Table 7.4, a twelfth instruction could be added:*

> 12. *Identify at least six topics that you had to know, use, and connect in order to successfully complete this assignment.*

This small addition encourages students to reflect on their integrative thinking, reinforcing the SCIL-OT principle that learning is not just about completing tasks, but about understanding how knowledge fits together into the logic of the profession.

Table 7.4 Occupational interview assignment illustrating the topic-to-topic connections required to complete successfully and a final question to get students to recognize their active connection-making process.

Interview assignment: instructions	
1. Identify an older adult with whom you know at least as an acquaintance—someone you would like to understand more as an occupational being.	◀ Humans as occupational beings (dynamics of occupation)
2. Decide how you will frame the interview for them and contact them to explain the purpose and invite them to participate and obtain their consent to record the interview.	◀ Explaining an occupational conversation in lay language ◀ Communication skills ◀ Consenting process
3. Using the occupational profile template, create questions that are conversational and open ended to gather information from the adult on their occupational history.	◀ Occupational profile (specific occupations) ◀ How the profile template relates to an interview ◀ Client-centered ◀ Active listening
4. Create open-ended, conversational questions about their current time use.	◀ Time use and occupation (specific and dynamics) ◀ Interview construction and implementation

Table 7.4 (Continued)

5. Determine how you will inquire about the meaning of their occupations over time and how the occupations have shaped the individual over time.	➤ How occupations generate (Dynamics of occupation): e.g., meaning, identity, social connections, self efficacy ➤ Translating topics into understandable questions
6. Determine how you will inquire about any occupational changes they face or fear as well as their occupational goals.	➤ Health risks associated with occupational losses (Dynamics of occupation) ➤ Resilience ➤ Volition
7. Determine how you will build rapport at the start of your time with the person.	➤ Communication ➤ Establishing safe environments ➤ Establishing rapport
8. Conduct the interview.	➤ Interview skills focused on occupation
9. Following the interview, analyze its content using the domains of the Occupational Therapy Practice Framework.	➤ Definitions of OTPF domains and how they present in a life
10. Identify the person's occupational supports and risks based on your how to listen for supports and risks, what constitutes supports and risks, why both supports and risks can exist together.	➤ How to listen for supports and risks, what constitutes supports and risks, why both supports and risks can exist together
11. Explain how and why an interview is one of occupational therapy's key practice tools.	➤ Knowledge of occupational therapy's distinctive purpose
12. **NEW:** Identify at least six topics you had to know, use, and connect in order to complete this assignment.	

Educators can similarly augment other written assignments to more fully engage students in topic-to-topic connection-making. Consider three common assignments in occupational therapy education:

- the *classic activity analysis*
- the *occupation analysis*
- the *case study*

Classic Activity Analysis

Early in their education, occupational therapy students often complete a classic activity analysis. Typically, they select a familiar activity and categorize it as self-care, work, play or leisure, or another domain. They may then analyze the activity across multiple dimensions—often guided by a professional document such as the Occupational Therapy Practice Framework (AOTA, 2020). After breaking the activity into as many aspects as possible, students may be asked to consider how the activity could be

- modified to accommodate an impairment.
- made more challenging to support capacity development.

To complete this assignment well, students must integrate numerous topics, such as the following:

- Dimensions of analysis (e.g., cultural, client factors)
- How impairments affect activity performance
- Adaptive strategies to optimize engagement

Occupation Analysis

This is a related assignment that parallels activity analysis but adds complexity. Students may observe someone engaged in occupation or videorecord themselves performing a familiar occupation. While many of the same topics apply, observing actual performance in context introduces additional layers, including the following:

- Observation skills
- Performance-related terminology
- Person–environment–occupation transactions
- Occupation as fluid and emergent
- Volition and subjective experience

- Personal assumptions about 'normal' performance—and the ability to bracket them
- The life context of the person observed
- How the occupation fits within roles, routines, and habits

Case Studies

While case studies serve many purposes, a frequent learning outcome is the development of professional reasoning. Students often identify and analyze the narrative, procedural, conditional, pragmatic, interactive, and sometimes ethical dimensions of reasoning that shape their understanding of the case. In doing so, they must connect numerous topics within and across each category. Often, though, assignments may not include requirements that actually make students aware of the interconnections they are making.

As educators, we design assignments like activity analyses, occupation analyses, and case studies because we want students to 'connect the dots.' We aim to create opportunities for students to experience how expert occupational therapists *think and act in dynamic, integrative ways*. Yet because topic integration is second nature to us as experts, we may forget that *students are still learning to see the connections* embedded in our assignments.

TIPS:

- *Ask students two to three times across the course to construct a concept map showing how they are connecting course units and topics from required readings.*
- *Encourage them to include selected topics from concurrent or previous courses.*
- *Afterward, share your own concept map and discuss similarities and differences in how each of you connects the topics.*
- *Consider using a prompt in several assignments like the one suggested earlier "Identify at least six topics that you had to know, use, and connect in order to successfully complete this assignment."*

These strategies help students visualize the intellectual architecture of the course, reinforcing the SCIL-OT Model's emphasis on integrative, subject-centered learning.

TOPIC-TO-TOPIC CONNECTION AT THE CLASSROOM LEVEL

Topics at the classroom level encompass both the topics students prepare for in advance and those that spontaneously emerge during class. Often by design, the key topics students encounter in preparatory materials—such as readings, study guides, or class schedules—resurface in the classroom through lectures and planned learning activities. Yet, due to the improvisational nature of teaching, new topics inevitably arise. Students ask questions, make comments, and bring in perspectives that introduce additional topics. Educators, in turn, respond by pulling in new ideas and connecting topics in new ways.

Topics at the classroom level therefore tend to expand and intermingle, often extending beyond those in the written materials. This expansion can enrich learning—but it can also become unproductive if not managed intentionally.

Whether tacitly or consciously, educators may expand classroom topics in ways that hinder student learning. One common scenario begins during class preparation. As we plan, our expert minds may start to think: How will students possibly understand topic X if I don't also include topics Y and Z? This reasoning leads us to introduce numerous additional topics beyond those students were prepared to engage with—potentially overwhelming them.

We may also inadvertently expand topics by dominating classroom time with lecture. In doing so, we presume that clear and repeated explanation will lead to understanding. Alternatively, we may allow student-introduced ideas—even those unrelated to the session's objectives—to dominate discussion. In either case, we risk relieving students of their own intellectual work: the effort required to comprehend, connect, and apply topics meaningfully to occupation.

To some degree, topic expansion is expected—and even desirable. Clarifying misunderstandings and deepening understanding often requires introducing new ideas. The classroom should help students contextualize and broaden the topics they encountered during preparation. But the key is this:

Educators must be selective and deliberate about which additional topics they bring forward.

We should focus only on those additional topics that help students deepen and contextualize their understanding of key ideas and their interconnections. In the classroom, we are challenged to help students identify and connect

- topics from the syllabus and preparatory materials.
- topics we selectively added for depth and breadth.
- relevant new topics that emerged spontaneously.

Our goal is to help students see that all these topics comprise a single, interconnected learning episode. In short, we help them create coherence—and we do so through intentional facilitation methods.

Three methods can help select and increase awareness of key topics, their interconnections, and their relationship to occupation:

1. Clear learning objectives for each class session
2. Class preparation guides for students
3. Class session guides for ourselves

Clear Learning Objectives

When writing *learning objectives for assignments*, we target the topic-to-topic connections we expect students to make. For example:

- Basic version of an intended learning outcome: demonstrate the ability to conduct an occupational performance observation assessment.
- Revised version: during an occupational performance observation assessment, evaluate supports and barriers to occupational engagement using clinical reasoning that connects theory, observation, performance skills, environmental elements, and task elements.

Class Preparation Guides

Guides may be given to students several days before class. These guides focus students' attention on the exact topics for class, their interconnections, and their relationship to occupation. They also:

- establish expectations that students will begin learning and connecting topics before class.
- signal that class time will build on—not repeat—preparatory work.

Table 7.5 Illustration of a class preparation guide highlighting questions that require students to make topic-to-topic connections.

Preparation guide questions (from assigned readings is assigned)	
As you read Chapter 1 in Radomski and Trombly, what sounds familiar in the first paragraph? Be specific about what content is pulled forward here from all your courses last semester.	◄ Students must connect topics across semesters
Carefully review the chapter's Case Example, with particular attention to the *reasoning of the OT*. Think back to the reasoning you used with the Colin case last semester. How does the OT reasoning compare and contrast to your reasoning with Colin? What do you already have practice thinking about from first semester? What from the reading will you need to add to what you think about in relation to clients' situations?	◄ Students must connect the expert's reasoning described in the text with their previous reasoning about a case. The connect topics to past and current experience and to self-assessment.
How is the OFM similar to or different from the top-down approach in the OTIPM?	◄ Question prompts students connect topics across readings

In other words, class is not a 're-do' of the readings in the instructor's words. It is a space for deepening and applying what students have already begun to learn and connect before class.

Excerpts from a class preparation guide for the first session of a course, *Enabling Occupation in Adulthood*, is presented in Table 7.5 with annotations on how the guide supports topic-to-topic connections.

Class Session Guide

A *class session guide* is a script that we, as educators, follow when implementing the class session. Box 7.2 presents a class session guide for a class that was held a couple of weeks after students completed the preparation guide in Table 7.5. The educator wrote himself specific instructions to follow and wording to use throughout the class session. While questioning is the primary linking strategy, slides, templates, role-plays, and other strategies are also used intentionally for connection-making.

BOX 7.2 SAMPLE CLASS PROCESS GUIDE ILLUSTRATING INTENTIONAL EMPHASIS ON TOPIC-TO-TOPIC CONNECTION MAKING

OT 543 Occupational Performance: Adult to Older Adult
Class Process Guide Week 3
8:00–8:10: Introduction to the session:

- Show slide with class learning outcomes. Remind students that the purpose of the outcomes is to give them a map of where they should steer their learning and where they should be at the end of class.
- **TIP:** *Show slide with the topics that students will work with in class today in order to achieve the outcomes*, for example, fieldwork experience, top-down assessment process, performance observation assessment, occupational analysis, motor skills, process skills, environmental supports and constraints, clinical reasoning, ROM, strength, sensation, endurance
- Show slide with the class agenda (the flow and timeline of activities taken from the process guide)

8:10–8:20: Touch base on fieldwork experiences this week. In small groups, discuss these questions:

- What did your FWE quiz you on this week?
- What resources did you use to look that up and explore the answer to that question in more depth afterward?
- What opportunities did you have to observe and demonstrate what you are learning about occupation and top-down approaches to practice?

  TIP: *Add this question to help students see how therapists they observed were linking many topics simultaneously: How did you see therapists using and connecting topics that we are addressing in this course so far?*

Transition by returning to the day's agenda on PPT.

8:20–9:00 Watch clips of Pam making cookies.

- Remind students that the video is starting in the middle of a larger assessment process. Ask: Given your knowledge of the OT assessment process, what did the OT likely do to get to this point in the assessment?

- In small groups, students establish the rationale for doing the performance observation assessment using cookies. Why would we as OTs take the time to create the opportunity and observe someone baking?
- During the video, complete the Occupation Analysis grid, determining steps of the performance and which steps students thought were a bit "sticky."
- Watch the performance again and complete the Motor/Process grid.
- Have students determine key (1) motor and process strengths; (2) motor and process challenges; and (3) environmental contributors to motor and process strengths and challenges
- Have students put it all together by using the script of "What I see is . . . What I think is . . . What I'd like to try next is . . . because . . ."

9:00–9:10 Break.

9:10 Transition: Use the graphics of the OFM and the OTIPM to show students where the above activities fall in the top-down process and where we go next.

9:15–9:40 Move further down the OFM and OTIPM models to the level of client factors:

- From the observation assessment, ask students: (1) What do we know about her upper extremity range of motion, strength, sensation and endurance? (2) What do you see that you want more information about? Why?

9:40–10:00 Have students do the assessment role-playing the decisions of what they would do next. Introduce and explain the assessment in relation to Pam's desired goals.

10:00–10:10 Break.

10:10–10:20 Have students identify the steps of the top-down assessment process they completed above.

10:20–10:40 Repeat the whole process with video of Virginia folding laundry.

10:40–10:55 Self-assessment.

- Have students briefly self-assess how well they met the learning outcomes for the day.

- **TIP:** *Have students identify all the topics they had to draw upon and connect in order to complete the day's learning activities. Which topics are becoming easier? Which were more challenging? What is their plan for revisiting the more challenging topics?*

10:55–11:00 Where we go from here in the next session; what topics we revisit and add.

TOPIC-TO-TOPIC CONNECTIONS AT THE PRACTICE EDUCATION LEVEL

Practice education inherently requires students to link multiple topics. At this level, topics are integral to the concepts, facts, theories, dispositions, and setting-specific procedures that we teach and model for students (see Figure 7.1). Topics are also embedded in the daily opportunities we create for students to observe, practice, apply, and demonstrate their learning in practice contexts.

Among many others, topics at the practice education level encompass a wide range of skills and concepts, including the following:

- Completing assessments
- Eliciting occupational profiles
- Receiving and applying feedback
- Modifying intervention plans based on client responses
- Teaching families
- Documenting services
- Coding and billing for services
- Handling ethical situations
- Communicating effectively with team members about occupational therapy's contributions, among many others

They also include client-specific considerations, such as clients' desired occupational goals, contextual supports and barriers, and procedures of particular practice settings.

While the core subject of occupation—its dynamics and specific forms—is prevalent across settings, the topics students must connect vary widely. What is essential in one setting may be peripheral in another. For example:

- In one setting, students may need to connect topics such as stroke, discharge planning, and assessments of client factors like range of motion, strength, tone, and balance.
- In another, they may need to connect anorexia, volition, mindfulness, and adolescence.

By identifying and connecting these complex, setting-specific topics to occupation, students learn to reason and create a path to optimize clients' occupational engagement. Yet expert practice educators often connect topics so naturally and fluidly that they may not recognize how many topics they are integrating in each situation. As a result, students may not appreciate the complexity of practice, because experts make it look seamless—and therefore deceptively simple.

Practice educators and Academic Fieldwork Coordinators (AFWCs) already use tools to help students process practice situations. For example:

- AFWCs often engage students through online discussion boards, where students report on clients, dilemmas, use of occupation, and other placement experiences.
- Practice educators often use weekly supervision meetings to discuss situations and help students see the full range of topics involved.

These tools can be extended to explicitly support connection-making. For instance, educators and AFWCs can use a conceptual model graphic to make topic connections visible. Students can use the graphic to map their reasoning—identifying all the topics related to a practice situation, how those topics influenced each other, and what actions they took as a result. Making their thinking explicit and visual allows students and educators to discuss overlooked topics and identify areas for further consideration.

Figure 7.2 illustrates a practice education experience in a community-based pain clinic, where occupational therapists used yoga to address pain and its effects, and to increase physical activity among people with chronic pain. The educator modified the SCIL-OT model graphic to map out the relevant topics and knowledge community for the setting. The graphic illustrated

- what resources students needed to locate and learn.
- with whom they needed to engage.

Students then created a portfolio organized by the topics and community members represented in the graphic. Most importantly, they had to anchor their learning and practice in the central idea that yoga—a specific occupation for some, an emerging occupation for others, and an activity for still others—was a means to manage pain and promote participation (dynamics of occupation)

The practice educator used the graphic to ask questions, guide discussions, and illustrate explanations, helping students identify and connect the topics needed to address clients' needs in this unique setting.

Similarly, a group of practice educators used the SCIL-OT graphic alongside a set of guiding questions to prepare for students arriving at their practice setting—and to reflect on their own teaching in the practice environment. These educators

- labeled members of the knowledge community with whom students would connect.
- identified priority topics students would need to learn and integrate.
- planned how they would help students learn "'on-the-lines"—that is, through the connections between topics, people, and occupations.

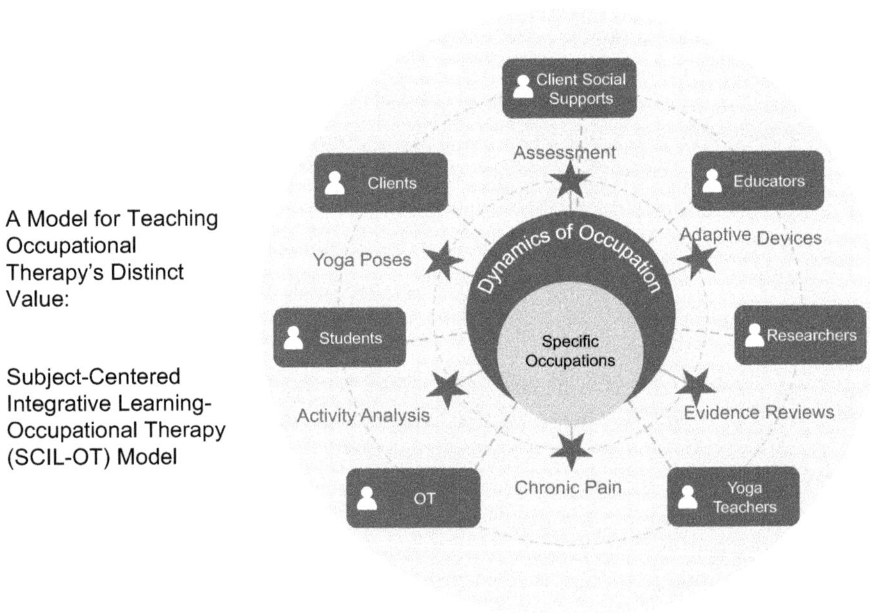

Figure 7.2 Students on placement label the SCIL-OT graphic to identify and connect topics important to providing service in a community setting.

Using prompts such as these, the practice educators created a subject-centered learning blueprint they could use when working with students:

- Explain how you will prompt students to link topics to specific occupations and to the dynamics of occupation.
- Explain how you will prompt students to connect to members of the knowledge community.
- Explain how you will prompt students to connect personally to occupation and empathize with those cut off from occupation.

In another example, a practice educator in a community-based day program for people with dementia used the SCIL-OT graphic as a pre- and post-session discussion tool. Having identified an occupational goal, exploring volunteer opportunities in the community, the educator and student

- labeled "Volunteer" under specific occupations.
- identified topics as the skills and resources the client would need to secure volunteer work.
- labeled members of the knowledge community as potential supports or challenges in achieving the goal.

This use of the SCIL-OT graphic helped students visualize the complexity of practice, anchoring their reasoning in the client's occupational goals and the broader context of the setting.

However, the SCIL-OT graphic is just one option for helping students connect topics to each other—and to occupation. A similar process can be used with the Canadian Model of Occupational Performance and Engagement (CMOP-E).

For example, the Canadian Model of Occupational Performance and Engagement (CMOP-E) can serve as an effective organizational frame. Educators can guide students to identify each component of the model in a given practice situation—such as the person, environment, and occupation—and then discuss how these components influence one another. In this framing:

- The occupation component parallels the SCIL-OT's focus on specific occupations.
- The person and environment components represent the kinds of topics students must learn to connect—such as volition, client factors, cultural context, or service delivery systems.

Using the CMOP-E in this way helps students visualize how topics interact to support or suppress occupational engagement. Like the coat rack metaphor, it provides a structure for organizing complex information and making meaningful connections

Using the CMOP-E, practice educators can ask students to

- identify each aspect of the model in a given practice situation.
- discuss how each aspect influences the others.

Regardless of the specific model selected, models serve as organizational frames and promote integrative learning, that is, topic-to-topic connections. They reduce cognitive overload, support reasoning, and help students connect topics to each other and to the central subject of occupation.

Metaphorically, imagine someone working in a coat check room at a theatre. Each patron drops off a coat. Without a system, the coat checker would quickly become overwhelmed with the number of individual coats. Fortunately, there's a rack with numbers and hooks, which provides a method to organize the coats. The rack relieves the burden of holding individual coats randomly and offers an orderly system—each coat is placed, labeled, and easily retrieved when needed.

Each strategy presented in this chapter functions like that coat rack system. Whether it's:

- a course description,
- a series of units in a course,
- an activity bridging one semester to the next,
- a class preparation guide,
- a class session guide, or
- a model mapping topics in practice education.

Each strategy is intentionally designed to help students recognize and know where to connect the current topics they are addressing. These frames support students in organizing their learning, making connections, and retrieving knowledge when needed—just as the coat rack helps the checker locate each coat.

Across the examples in this chapter, the key to helping students connect topics—whether at the curriculum, course, class, or practice education level—is providing an organizational frame. An organizational frame shows students where individual topics fit within a larger schema of knowledge. It gives students a way to make sense of topics, offering a mental structure for how to file each one in relation to others.

TIP: *It is important, however, that educators help students go beyond merely attaching elements of the situation to the categories of an organizational frame. Students must also be required to explain how topics mutually influence each other—and how they, in transaction, support or suppress occupational engagement. This kind of mapping makes integrative reasoning visible and teachable, reinforcing the SCIL-OT Model's emphasis on learning through connection-making.*

Use the following self-assessment tool to review how explicitly your materials and learning processes guide students to make topic-to-topic connections. This tool prompts a simple, intuitive reflection on how strongly students are able—or are asked—to make topic-to-topic connections at four levels:

- Curriculum
- Course
- Class session
- Practice education

CURRICULUM DESIGN ACTIVITY: EVALUATING AND STRENGTHENING TOPIC-TO-TOPIC CONNECTION MAKING

The following exercise may be completed individually or collaboratively with other members of the faculty group. It supports ongoing refinement of teaching practices aligned with the SCIL-OT Model's emphasis on integrative, subject-centered learning.

The lines represent a continuum from Weak to Strong.

- **At the Weak end:** Students are not explicitly and consistently asked to identify how they are connecting topics to other topics.
- **At the Strong end:** Students are explicitly and consistently asked to identify how they are connecting topics to other topics.
- **In the middle:** Topics are intentionally designed to connect, yet students may or may not be aware of the connections constructed by faculty and practice educators.

Instructions:

- Rate the strength of topic-to-topic connection-making at each level of your teaching by marking an X on the continuum between Weak and Strong.
- Then, identify three ways topic-to-topic connection-making could be strengthened at each level.

Note: Suggestions for strengthening may be minor but impactful. For example:

- Add a question to class preparation materials asking students to specifically relate the session's topics to the prior session's topics, or
- Add an instruction to the assignment: Identify at least six topics you had to know, use, and connect in order to complete this assignment, or
- Revise rubrics to assess students' ability to connect topics to each other and to occupation.

Small changes like these can have a substantial impact.

Large-Content Program Topics Connect to Vision, Mission, Philosophy

Weak —————————————————— Strong

Three suggestions to strengthen connections at the program level:

1.
2.
3.

Course Materials and Assignments Emphasize Making Topic-to-Topic Connections

Weak —————————————————— Strong

Three suggestions to strengthen topic-to-topic connections at the course level:

1.
2.
3.

Class Session Processes Emphasize Making Topic-to-Topic Connections

Weak —————————————————— Strong

Three suggestions to strengthen topic-to-topic connections at the class session level:

1.
2.
3.

Practice Education Emphasizes Making Topic-to-Topic Connections

Weak Strong

Three suggestions to strengthen topic-to-topic connections during practice education:

1.
2.
3.

CONCLUSION

The main idea of Chapter 7 is that we, as educators, intentionally create educational processes that emphasize the interdependence of topics—their mutual influences and their relationships to occupation. This principle holds true regardless of the curriculum level we are focused on: whether designing a full program, structuring a course, planning a class session, or guiding students in practice education.

By guiding students to consciously connect multiple topics to one another—and to the core subject of occupation—we create strong and explicit coherence across all levels of the curriculum. This coherence supports integrative reasoning, deepens understanding, and prepares students to think and act as occupational therapists who recognize the complexity and interconnectedness of human engagement.

REFERENCES

American Occupational Therapy Association. (2020). *Occuaptional Therapy Practice Framework: Domain and process* (4th ed.). Author.

American Occupational Therapy Association. (2021). Occupational therapy curriculum design framework. *American Journal of Occupational Therapy*, *75*(Suppl. 3). https://doi.org/10.5014/ajot.2021.75S3008

Chapter 8

Connecting Students to a Knowledge Community

INTRODUCTION

As introduced in Chapter 4, the SCIL-OT Model upholds the principle that 'it takes a village' to learn and develop knowledge and skills related to the dynamics by which occupation affects health and well-being, and how therapists enable health- and well-being-supporting occupational engagement. The metaphorical village represents the diverse community of people with whom students interact to develop these understandings. Thus, the term knowledge community refers to everyone in a particular context who is a resource for learning. Members of the knowledge community, represented by the rectangles and human icons in Figure 8.1, are resources for learning about the dynamics of occupation, specific occupations, enabling occupation, and also the various topics students must connect to occupation.

Members of the knowledge community variously include researchers and authors, interprofessional colleagues, educators, students, clients, and others in the client's constellation of social supports. Who constitutes the knowledge community shifts across courses and learning experiences. The knowledge community for a program development course, for example, may include community sites with whom the program has a relationship, leaders in occupational therapy who work in program development, peer colleagues, and faculty. The knowledge community for a course on the occupations of childhood may include children, parents, and day-care centers where students may observe children at play.

Similarly, the configuration of the knowledge community varies across practice contexts. In a school setting, for example, the knowledge community includes occupational therapists and students, teachers, children and their families, social workers, principals, and school counselors, among others. In a hospital setting, it includes occupational therapists and students, physicians, nurses, patients and

DOI: 10.4324/9781003635628-10

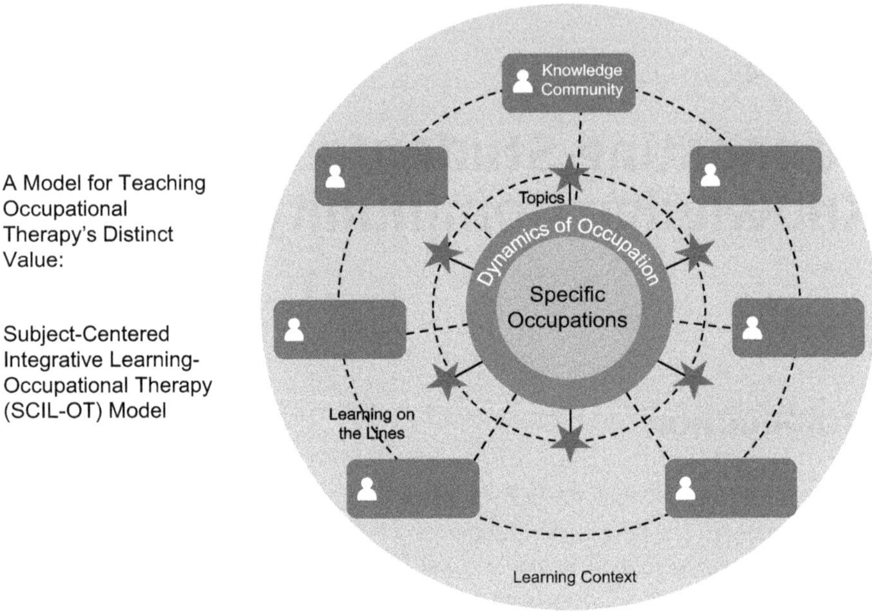

Figure 8.1 The knowledge community is represented by the outer ring of linked rectangles.

their social supports, and interprofessional colleagues who may differ from those with whom students would engage in a school or other community setting.

While the presence of a knowledge community is constant, its members change with each setting and educational experience. Yet, students and educators alike may not always recognize these engagements as participation in a knowledge community. It is vital, therefore, that we, as educators, design educational experiences that explicitly draw students' attention to the process of actively constructing knowledge with—and through interactions with—members of various knowledge communities across their education.

Therefore, in this chapter, we first explore how designing a knowledge community includes—but also goes beyond—typical practices like inviting guest lecturers, designating people and organizations in the community for students to visit, or creating interprofessional experiences. To design knowledge communities intentionally, we must carefully select members based on their strong alignment with—and potential contributions to—the learning objectives of our program, its courses, class sessions, and approaches to practice education.

Additionally, designing knowledge communities involves putting in place instructional supports that enhance students' interactions with community members and help them expand the meaning of those interactions. After these explanations, we provide design activities, illustrations, and tips that educators can use to assemble an intentional knowledge community as a key component of students' learning experiences.

OBJECTIVES

This chapter will help educators to:

1. Design learning opportunities that connect students to diverse knowledge communities with emphasis on co-constructing knowledge.
2. Identify and differentiate what constitutes knowledge communities across the four component areas of a curriculum: the education program, the courses, the classroom, and practice education.
3. Assess and strengthen connection-making to knowledge communities across the four component areas of a curriculum.

DESIGNING CONNECTIONS TO KNOWLEDGE COMMUNITIES EXTENDS BEYOND ACQUIRING CONTENT AND INTERPERSONAL SKILLS

There is already a strong tradition in occupational therapy education of connecting students with members of the local knowledge community. Educators, for example, connect students with clients, families, and interprofessional colleagues. Educators connect students to each other through small group discussion and projects, and we foster the educator-student connection through mentorship and coaching. We connect students to relevant community organizations and services. We also connect students to researchers and leaders in the field through textbook selection, visiting lectureships, and assigned readings. All the ways that educators connect students to others was the basis for naming relational learning as one of the signature pedagogies in occupational therapy (Schaber, 2014).

Educators often view these connections as opportunities for students to acquire content and develop interpersonal skills. Students engage with peers, clients, interprofessional colleagues, and people different from themselves to develop communication skills, engage in therapeutic use of self, practice interviewing skills, create occupational profiles, discover community resources, and learn the roles and responsibilities of other professions. Similarly, students engage with assigned authors and guest lecturers to acquire certain concepts and skills.

When applying the SCIL-OT Model, we intentionally engage three processes that move these interactions beyond acquiring content and skills.

The first process involves intentionally selecting and assembling the people with whom students will interact. We select these members based on how they might help students learn to notice, understand, and experience the dynamics of occupation, specific occupations, and how various topics relate to occupation. As illustrated in Table 8.1, each member of the knowledge community has information, experiences, and perspectives that can illuminate students' understandings of occupation and related topics.

The second process begins to shift the focus of these interactions from acquiring content to how students are actively constructing knowledge about occupation and its relationship to health and well-being. This step often requires supplemental

Table 8.1 Sample members of the knowledge community and what students can learn from members' experience and expertise.

Members of the knowledge community	What students can learn about occupation and related topics
Researchers and scholars	Conceptual and empirical understandings, terminology, and critical perspectives of the dynamics of occupation and specific occupations. Evidence related to topics students are learning.
Clients and families	Narrative understandings of specific occupations, how the dynamics of occupation are present in occupational engagement, and the myriad ways an occupation is performed and experienced in response to specific contexts.
Educators	Same as above, plus how disparate topics relate to the dynamics of occupation and specific occupations.
Interprofessional colleagues	Related knowledge that supports students' occupation knowledge; what knowledge of occupation adds to a care team.
Other learners	Contribute prior, diverse experiences with occupation and new understandings emerging through their educational experiences.

instructional processes like those described in the next section of this chapter. This support is needed for several reasons. As many educators have experienced, merely having students interact with others (for instance, in a small group discussion) does not automatically result in new understandings or knowledge among group members. Moreover, on their own, most students are unlikely to tune into processes of knowledge construction. Many students are also unlikely (as discussed in Chapter 3) to perceive themselves as knowledge creators.

Hence, guided by the SCIL-OT Model, educators design instructional processes that engage students in co-constructing, with other members of a knowledge community, knowledge about key content areas—including occupation, the relationship of occupation to health and well-being, how various topics relate to occupation, and how to enable occupational engagement. To ensure focused inquiry into these key content areas, we supplement students' interactions with intentional prompts, guiding questions, discussion objectives, and expectations for reporting. We also explicitly draw students' attention to the new understandings and knowledge they have created, as well as to their processes of knowledge creation.

The third process involves drawing students' attention to parallels between how they construct new knowledge through their engagements with knowledge communities in the academic program and how occupational therapists around the world likewise create and revise new knowledge for the profession broadly in and through practice. We therefore intentionally use various learning activities, assignments, and assessments that help students comprehend that their 'doings' in their own knowledge communities mirror the processes by which the profession itself evolves. In other words, we help students comprehend that—whether on local or profession-wide levels—knowledge is co-constructed through communal observing, dialoguing, debating, comparing and contrasting, refining, researching, synthesizing, translating, drawing and justifying new conclusions, and seeing things in a new light. The hope, therefore, is that by engaging with members of a knowledge community, students experience themselves as participants in an ongoing process of knowledge construction and develop professional identities as active creators of knowledge.

In sum, the emphasis given to knowledge communities in the SCIL-OT Model points to three processes:

1. Selecting the people with whom students will interact.
2. Supplementing students' interactions with instructional processes that engage them explicitly in co-constructing knowledge about occupation, its relation to health and well-being, how various topics relate to occupation, and enabling occupational engagement.

3. Drawing students' attention to the fact that their co-construction of knowledge mirrors how knowledge is constructed in the profession at large.

In following these processes, we, as educators, must seek to ensure that all members of knowledge communities—not only our students—benefit in some way, especially actual clients, persons in the client's constellations, members of underserved and underrepresented groups, or community-based service organizations. To help ensure mutual benefit, we help students learn that engagement involves understanding and respecting the situations and experiences of those with whom they engage. We help them learn that engagement involves awareness of colonialist assumptions and biases about learning from others. We show them that engagement involves entering all relationships in learning and practice contexts from a stance of intellectual humility, collaboration, and openness to the unique subjectivities and experiences of others.

The next section provides activities, illustrations, and tips that can facilitate infusing these processes into student learning experiences at the program, course, class, and practice education levels.

DESIGNING KNOWLEDGE COMMUNITY CONNECTIONS AT THE PROGRAM LEVEL

At the program level, selecting the people who constitute the students' knowledge community is driven by the program's vision, philosophy, aims, and institutional context. Educators may, for example, select as members of the knowledge community the faculty group, interdisciplinary scholars in the institution, and specific local and regional external partners. A program that has a particular theoretical model as its framework—such as Enabling Occupation, the Person-Environment-Occupation-Performance model, or Transactionalism—will also select authors who write about these models as members of students' program-level knowledge community. These selections reflect and reinforce the program's vision, philosophy, aims, and context.

The vision, mission, philosophy, aims, and context of the curriculum are, of course, infused across the entire program. Therefore, members selected for the knowledge community at the program level are linked to those selected at the course, class, and even placement levels. Some may be carried forward across all levels, such as the program faculty or particular external partners. At the program level, however, the focus is on selecting members of students' knowledge community who support the overall curriculum design. These members can be identified and nurtured using the instructional design activities and tips below.

Tips For Assembling Program-Level Knowledge Communities (Boxes 8.1–8.3)

TIP 1: *Explore Local Expertise and Lived Experience*

Ask who in this institution or community is doing work—or has lived experience—that relates to the dynamics of occupation, specific occupations, or the key topics emphasized in the curriculum?

TIP 2: *Scan Internal and External Contexts*

Look for individuals, programs, and organizations whose work aligns with occupational therapy concepts, even if they don't use occupational language. Examples include scholars studying everyday living, service-learning initiatives, creative arts and health programs, and campus makers' labs.

TIP 3: *Wrap Topic-Specific Expertise in Instructional Processes*

When engaging someone whose expertise isn't explicitly occupational, design learning activities that guide students to connect the topic to the dynamics of occupation.

Example: In a splinting session, ask students to identify how the splint supports or hinders occupational performance, and how it might affect sleep and well-being.

BOX 8.1 CURRICULUM DESIGN ACTIVITY TO SCAN THE ENVIRONMENT TO DISCOVER POTENTIAL MEMBERS OF STUDENTS' KNOWLEDGE COMMUNITY AT THE PROGRAM LEVEL

Begin by reviewing key elements of your curriculum design—such as the program's vision, mission, philosophy, aims, threads, and outcomes. Then, scan your institutional and community contexts for potential knowledge community members who align with these elements. Consider the following sources:

- Curriculum vitae posted on websites of other professions, disciplines, and centers within your department, division, school, or college

  Example: Faculty affiliated with your institution's Center on Aging, Master of Public Health program, Human Development program, Construction Management, or Disability Studies

- Flyers and email announcements about upcoming presentations at your institution

  Example: A Disability Studies scholar presenting on caregiving; a Psychology panel on meaning in life; a student-led discussion on universal design and accessibility

- Promotions of new initiatives featured in institutional news blasts

  Example: A collaboration between engineering and design students to create clothing for children with disabilities

- Departmental newsletters highlighting faculty publications

  Example: Physical therapy faculty publishing on telehealth or psychosocial factors in chronic pain

- Faculty expertise repositories maintained by your institution

  Example: Humanities or social science faculty whose research intersects with occupational therapy themes

- Institutional programs and services that support occupational engagement

  Example: Programs for first-generation college students or students on the autism spectrum transitioning to college

- Local organizations that address occupational engagement

  Example: Groups focused on affordable housing, food access, aging in place, transportation, or employment for underserved populations

- Occupational therapy practice sites that reflect the program's philosophy and aims

REFLECTION PROMPT

- What surprised you in this scan?
- What new partnerships, learning opportunities, or knowledge community connections might emerge from these discoveries?

BOX 8.2 CURRICULUM DESIGN ACTIVITY TO EVALUATE EXISTING PARTNERS AS KNOWLEDGE COMMUNITY MEMBERS AND STRENGTHEN ALIGNMENT OF THEIR CONTRIBUTIONS WITH THE CURRICULUM

If you are in an established program, you have in place a robust knowledge community but may not have framed it as such for students. Additionally, some members have likely been sustained in the knowledge community out of tradition. Certain lecturers may be popular with students so they are invited back year after year even though their specific contribution may no longer be clear or may be askew to a newly revised curriculum. An annual event with a community organization may remain popular but the learning purpose may have faded. Take a moment here to review the significant members of the knowledge community already within your program who support students' learning. Consider completing a table following the example below:

List the program's key partners	Intended learning contribution	Are the learning contributions clear?		How to strengthen connections to occupation through interactions with this knowledge community member
		To students?	To the partner?	
e.g., local chapter of organization supporting and advocating for the transgender community	Understand the range of lived experiences of people in LGBTQIA+ community, the relationship between sexual identities and occupation, the impact of bias and policy on occupational engagement,	Most students love this panel each year; some find it troubling due to their beliefs. Purpose of the panel is not as explicit as it could be to students.	We have invited this group for several years but have not communicated our interest in how everyday occupations shape and are shaped by experiences of sexual identities.	- Design a preparatory activity that will set the stage and make clear to students why we hold this event.

(Continued)

	the role of occupation in confronting bias, understand occupational needs, supports, barriers the community faces.			- Set a climate that is inclusive and safe for panel members to share their life experiences. Let them know how their experiences relate to students' understandings of occupation. - Ask students to reflect on how bias, stigma, and policy can disable meaningful engagement.
e.g., first-year design students in engineering	Students learn engineering perspectives on solving problems related to participation in health-related activities; Students share occupational perspectives with interprofessional colleagues; OT students contribute knowledge of the P–E–O transaction to design.	Yes	Yes	In addition to completing the product, ask students to compare and contrast engineering and occupational therapy perspectives, identify what an OT perspective offers to designing products to help people, explain that perspective, explain what an engineering perspective adds to OT . . .

(Continued)

e.g., annual event with local prosthetics vendors	Introduce students to a broad array of prosthetics and companies.	Yes, in relation to prosthetics—how they work, how to get them on/off, etc. but less so in terms of occupation.	Yes, in relation to the topic of prosthetics	Observe people performing specific occupations while wearing the prosthesis, analyze how the environment relates to successful prosthetic use; examine when prosthetics enable occupation and when they disable occupational engagement and why.

Identifying members of the knowledge community whose contributions have faded in relevance to the curriculum does not mean that those members necessarily need to be dropped. It may mean simply that a review of the focus of the partnership may need to be revisited and instructional processes created to make the purpose explicit. It may also mean that educators help members of the knowledge community modify their engagements to align more strongly with the curriculum design.

Sometimes members of the knowledge community are included because of the program's unique location, institutional context, or history. For example, your program may be situated in a region seeking reparation and representation for Indigenous Peoples. In such cases, you might choose to emphasize the impact of injustice on occupation—and conversely, how occupation can be a source for reducing inequities.

To support this emphasis, you would cultivate a knowledge community that includes students and faculty who are members of Indigenous Peoples groups, researchers who partner with Indigenous Peoples communities, individuals who identify as Indigenous Peoples, and community organizations working toward justice for Indigenous Peoples.

This knowledge community, shaped by the program's context, should influence the program's philosophy statement, content, courses, and learning experiences. For example:

- The philosophy statement might include a commitment to Indigenous Peoples.
- The curriculum might include content and threads related to culture–injustice–occupation transactions.
- The program's rituals, such as graduation or orientation, might include elements honoring Indigenous Peoples.

BOX 8.3 CURRICULUM DESIGN ACTIVITY TO CREATE CONTINUITY BETWEEN THE KNOWLEDGE COMMUNITY AND ELEMENTS OF THE CURRICULUM DESIGN

1. *List the distinct members of students' knowledge community* with whom the program partners because of its distinctive context.
2. *Review the following curriculum design elements* and determine whether the knowledge community—and the program's focus shaped by those key members—is adequately reflected in each:
   a. Vision
   b. Mission
   c. Curriculum Threads
   d. Program Outcomes
   e. Philosophy Statement
   f. Courses
   g. Content

DESIGNING KNOWLEDGE COMMUNITY CONNECTIONS AT THE COURSE LEVEL

It is likely that each course—and even each unit or module—will have its own distinct knowledge community. This includes the authors selected for the course, invited participants, individuals who students contact for assignments, the instructor, and the students themselves. Designing a course-level knowledge community involves both selecting the people with whom students will engage and creating instructional processes that highlight connections to occupation and the knowledge construction that occurs through those engagements (Box 8.4).

BOX 8.4 CURRICULUM DESIGN ACTIVITY—FOUR STEPS FOR INTENTIONALLY ASSEMBLING AND ORIENTING THE KNOWLEDGE COMMUNITY FOR A COURSE

STEP 1: CLARIFY THE COURSE'S RELATIONSHIP TO OCCUPATION

Whether your course focuses directly or indirectly on occupation, revisit why it is important to students' understanding of occupation as a factor in health and well-being. This clarity will guide the prompts you create in Step 3 and how you prepare guests in Step 4.

Instructions: Write a brief explanation of how the course and its topics relate to the dynamics of occupation and occupational engagement. Consider sharing this with students or incorporating it into the course description.

Reflect: How does this course relate to occupation and health/well-being?

STEP 2: IDENTIFY MEMBERS OF THE KNOWLEDGE COMMUNITY

Use the tables below to list members of the knowledge community based on the course's focus and learning outcomes.

A. Based on course focus areas

Focus area in the course	Members of the Knowledge Community with whom students will interact around that focus area	Purpose of the interaction/ contribution to understanding the topic and relation to occupation

B. Based on course outcomes

Outcome for the course	Members of the knowledge community with whom students will interact to support the outcome	Purpose of the interaction in advancing the outcome

Reflect: Does the purpose of the interaction include the content focus, its relationship to occupation, and its relationship to health and well-being?

STEP 3: CREATE PROMPTS TO SUPPORT KNOWLEDGE CONSTRUCTION

Students may enjoy guest lectures or field visits, but enjoyment alone doesn't guarantee learning. Help students connect these experiences to their growing understanding of occupation and recognize their role in constructing knowledge through community engagement.

A. Prompts to connect content to occupation

List three simple prompts that help students link the topic to occupation and health/well-being.

Example: Free-write a one-minute paper explaining at least two ways today's topic adds to your understanding of occupation.

1. ____
2. ____
3. ____

B. Prompts to highlight knowledge construction

List three prompts that help students recognize how they are constructing knowledge.

Example: List three things you did with today's content (compare, contrast, connect) that took it beyond what you heard or experienced.

1. ______________________________
2. ______________________________
3. ______________________________

C. Prompts to connect to the profession's knowledge-creation practices

List three prompts that help students see how their learning mirrors how the profession constructs knowledge.

Example: Share your free-write in a group of three. Ask each other to clarify unclear points and revise your writing based on the dialogue.

1. ______________________________
2. ______________________________
3. ______________________________

STEP 4: PREPARE MEMBERS OF THE KNOWLEDGE COMMUNITY

When planning student engagements, communicate with members of the knowledge community about the aims of the interaction. Include both content outcomes and outcomes related to students' ability to link the interaction to occupation and occupational engagement.

Briefly outline what you will share with each guest to help them understand their role in supporting students' learning about occupation.

DESIGNING KNOWLEDGE COMMUNITY CONNECTIONS AT THE CLASS SESSION LEVEL

As noted in Chapter 6, designing each class session involves creating a subset of intended learning outcomes for the day that align with the overall course objectives. These daily outcomes help determine the session's topics—and together, they guide the selection of a knowledge community for that class session.

Authors, guest lecturers, peer learning activities, and community members are selected based on how they advance students' understanding of the topic. For example:

- A class on occupational therapy in acute care may include a panel of therapists working in that context.
- A class on joint replacements may feature a lecture by an orthopedic surgeon.
- A session on transfers may engage students with each other as they practice different types of transfers.

What's important about these interactions is that students take the content from the engagement and create links to the core concepts of occupation, health, and well-being.

The design process at the class session level mirrors the process used at the course level:

1. Consider the learning outcomes and topics for the session.
2. Select and design the interactions students will have to reinforce the learning outcomes.
3. Prompt students to make connections between those interactions and enabling occupational engagement.
4. Encourage students to recognize that their connection-making is part of co-constructing knowledge.

One feature that shifts slightly at the class session level is that instructors and peers play a more prominent role in the knowledge community.

BOX 8.5 END OF CLASS WRAP-UP ILLUSTRATING PROMPTS TO GUIDE STUDENTS' ATTENTION TO THE KNOWLEDGE CONSTRUCTION PROCESS THAT OCCURRED IN CLASS AND A CONNECTION BACK TO OCCUPATION

Class session topic: Wheelchair transfers and mobility

"Today we've been learning the skill of helping people move from one place to another in their environment. The knowledge community with whom we've been constructing these skills includes your peers, me as your instructor, our guests, the authors you read for class, and the people you watched in the videos."

"With two of your peers, take five minutes to respond to these prompts:"

1. List the knowledge and skills you constructed through input from each member of the knowledge community—your peers, instructor, authors, video participants, and guests. How did you take input from all these sources and create new understandings for yourself today?
2. How do your new understandings and skills relate to occupation as a source of health and well-being and to enabling occupational engagement?

DESIGNING KNOWLEDGE COMMUNITY CONNECTIONS AT THE PRACTICE EDUCATION LEVEL

When students begin their practice education placements, educators typically orient them to the setting by having them observe how occupational therapists engage with clients and families. Students may also be asked to interview and shadow members of the interprofessional team and observe team communications. Through these experiences, students learn the roles and responsibilities of occupational therapists in the setting, how to communicate with different team members, and how the team engages clients in the therapy process.

As students begin to engage with clients, families, and interprofessional colleagues, they naturally become members of the team. However, this participation is not always framed as engagement in a knowledge community. Upon closer examination, the team's collaborative work—assessing clients, communicating, and planning interventions—is a process of constructing shared understandings about client needs and how to support them.

Occupational therapy students contribute to this process by sharing their assessment findings and disciplinary perspectives. Practice educators can help students reframe their participation as co-constructing knowledge with others. This reframing can be supported through the following three approaches.

TIP 1: *Prompt Students to Share Occupational Insights*

Encourage students to explain—both verbally and in writing—how their assessment data relates to clients' specific occupations and the role those occupations play in overall health and well-being. These prompts remind students that they contribute occupation-specific knowledge to the team's collective understanding.

In SCIL-OT language, educators prompt students to engage with the knowledge community on-the-line between assessment/intervention topics and the core subject of occupation.

TIP 2: *Address Power Dynamics Around Knowledge*

Help students recognize and navigate power issues that can arise in interprofessional teams. Students may lack confidence in their own knowledge and defer to others—especially when medical knowledge is prioritized. Educators can

- observe when students mimic others' knowledge to fit in.
- discuss how certain settings may unintentionally devalue occupational knowledge.
- explore whether students feel pressure to downplay their focus on occupation or overemphasize medical knowledge.

These conversations help students question whose knowledge is valued and empower them to advocate for the relevance of occupational knowledge in collaborative care.

TIP 3: *Clarify Disciplinary Distinctions*

Students may feel confused when multiple professions address similar client-related topics—such as activities of daily living, home safety, or cognition. Using the

SCIL-OT Model, educators can help students see that while many professions share concerns about these topics, each links them to different disciplinary subjects.

What makes occupational therapy distinctive is how it connects these shared topics to the core subject of occupation. The activity in Box 8.6 illustrates one way to help students make this connection.

BOX 8.6 CURRICULUM DESIGN ACTIVITY USING THE SCIL-OT MODEL GRAPHIC TO GUIDE STUDENT SUPERVISION/COACHING MEETING ON PLACEMENT

Chapter 7 included an illustration of students using the SCIL-OT model graphic to map the topics addressed in a placement setting. Here, students continue that practice by adding to the graphic the members of the knowledge community in the placement setting. Consider the following steps during a supervision meeting.

1. Ask students to bring to the supervision meeting the SCIL-OT graphic on which they mapped the topics addressed in the setting.
2. Using the same graphic, ask students to assign each of the outer rectangles of the graphic to a member of the knowledge community such as, in a school setting, a particular child, particular teachers, the family, specific interprofessional colleagues, other children, the principal, and others. Be sure students do not forget to include themselves in the circle.
3. Going further, ask students to draw a line from each member of the knowledge community to the topics each addresses in the setting. Each member of the community may address aspects of several topics.
4. Ask students to explain if and how each member of the knowledge community contributes to their knowledge of one of the topics.
5. Ask the student to further explain how they take their expanding topic knowledge and relate it to the dynamics of occupation, generally, and also to specific occupations.
6. Have the student explain how they contribute distinctive knowledge of the topic to the team because of their knowledge and perspective of occupation.
7. Reinforce that most topics are not the exclusive domain of a single member of the knowledge community. Their distinctive contribution to the knowledge community comes from how they connect shared topics to the core of occupation.

CURRICULUM DESIGN ACTIVITY: EVALUATING AND STRENGTHENING STUDENT-TO-KNOWLEDGE COMMUNITY CONNECTIONS

The following exercise may be completed individually or collaboratively with other members of the faculty group. It supports ongoing refinement of teaching practices aligned with the SCIL-OT Model's emphasis on integrative, subject-centered learning.

The lines represent a continuum from Weak to Strong.

- **At the Weak end:** Program documents do not explicitly and consistently address the knowledge community or its purpose in the curriculum OR Students are not explicitly and consistently required to notice their role in constructing knowledge through their interactions.
- **At the Strong end:** Program documents clearly and robustly address the knowledge community and its purpose in the curriculum OR Students are explicitly and consistently required to connect to members of the knowledge community and to notice their role as knowledge creators.
- **In the middle:** Student-to-knowledge community connections are present but may remain part of the instructors' background rationale in course designs or may not be integrated into how students are assessed.

Instructions:

- Rate the strength of knowledge community connection-making at each level of your program or teaching by marking an X on the continuum between Weak and Strong.
- Then, identify three ways knowledge community connection-making could be strengthened at each level, including students' awareness of their role as knowledge co-creators in the community.

Note: Suggestions for strengthening may be minor but impactful. For example:

- Add a question to class preparation materials asking students to specifically name how they assembled knowledge across the readings to answer questions, or
- Add an instruction to an assignment.
- Revise rubrics to assess students' ability to explain their role in knowledge co-creation with others.

Small changes like these can have a substantial impact.

Knowledge Community Connections in Key Curriculum Documents (Vision, Mission, Philosophy)

Weak ———————————————— **Strong**

Three suggestions to strengthen connections at the program level:

1.
2.
3.

Course Materials and Assignments Emphasize Knowledge Community Connections

Weak ———————————————— **Strong**

Three suggestions to strengthen connections at the course level:

1.
2.
3.

Class Session Processes Emphasize Making Knowledge Community Connections

Weak ———————————————— **Strong**

Three suggestions to strengthen connections at the class session level:

1.
2.
3.

Practice Education Emphasizes Knowledge Community Connections

Weak ———————————————— **Strong**

Three suggestions to strengthen connections during practice education:

1.
2.
3.

CONCLUSION

When students enter our educational programs, they enter the process of becoming members of knowledge communities who actively co-construct knowledge. Students, however, do not necessarily recognize yet that they are co-constructing knowledge with others. Therefore, as educators we select instructional processes that bring them into relationship with others and that highlight the knowledge-making process they engage in through those relationships. For example, when students interview others or compile an occupational profile, we prompt them to identify how the interview added to their understanding of how occupation works in human lives or why specific occupations can have different meanings in different situations. When we assign a reading about the Model of Human Occupation (Kielhofner, 2008), we frame the readings as not only learning about the model but also actively engaging with Kielhofner and others through their writings to construct knowledge of occupation and its relationships to health and well-being. We ask students what contributions they would like to make to Kielhofner's representations of occupation. In these examples, we help students see themselves as participating in community to build knowledge.

Intentionally connecting students to knowledge communities is grounded in the principle that knowledge is communal; knowledge is continuously generated, evaluated, and revised among people in interaction with each other and with constantly changing situations (Palmer, 2017). Good teaching, therefore, replicates "the process of knowing by engaging students in the dynamics" of the knowledge community (p. 115). The knowledge community gathers around a great thing that exists in the world in order to explore it, generate tentative understandings of it, evaluate those understandings in light of new learning, and overtime revise those understandings. The great thing in occupational therapy is occupation and how occupation, health, and well-being interact. Exploring this great thing, occupational therapy knowledge communities in and across various sociocultural contexts construct histories, generate data, consider multiple perspectives, create theory, engage in debate, apply current understandings to real-world needs, and remain open to emerging understandings. Therefore, connecting students to knowledge communities refers to replicating this process of knowing so that students take their seat as members of the knowledge community who assemble, translate, and apply knowledge of occupation. To replicate the knowledge community does not require "that we put the chairs in a circle and have a conversation" (Palmer, 2017, p. 115). Connecting students to the knowledge community is a principle that educators can realize through numerous instructional processes, including lectures, labs, simulation, capstones, service-learning, problem-based learning, and others. The point is that whatever instructional process is used, it is designed to draw students' attention to how the field creates knowledge of occupation and related knowledge and to their engagement in the process.

REFERENCES

Kielhofner, G. (2008). *Model of human occupation: Theory and application*. Lippincott Williams & Wilkins.

Palmer, P. J. (2017). *The courage to teach: Exploring the inner landscape of a teacher's life*. John Wiley & Sons.

Schaber, P. (2014). Searching for and identifying signature pedagogies in occupational therapy education. *American Journal of Occupational Therapy*, *68*, S40–S44. https://doi.org/10.5014/ajot.2014.685S08

Chapter 9

The Significance of Reimagining

Occupation-Centered Curricula

INTRODUCTION

Designing Occupation-Centered Curricula and Instruction for Occupational Therapy Students is the culmination of years of learning about how we and many other educators might successfully design, implement, evaluate, and improve upon occupation-centered education. In writing this book, we imagined that many educators have discovered, as we certainly have, that the work of realizing and strengthening occupation-centered education is challenging, ongoing, and deeply meaningful.

The work of occupation-centered education is not prescriptive or formulaic. It does not follow a set of definitive steps or processes. It goes beyond offering a series of lectures, labs, or courses on occupation. Instead, it requires educators to continuously design and redesign learning experiences that center occupation as the core subject.

This work is complex, evolving, and transformative. It is never truly finished and must permeate every layer of educational design—from the program level to each course, individual class session, and practice education experience. And because it is always in motion, it invites educators to remain reflective, adaptive, and committed to improvement.

Chapter 9 serves several purposes in support of this ongoing work. First, we offer a concise synopsis of key principles and guidelines from the SCIL-OT Model. Second, we explore how educators might use the SCIL-OT Model in conjunction with other curriculum and learning design approaches to enhance occupation-centered education. Lastly, we encourage new schema for organizing knowledge in occupational therapy curricula.

DOI: 10.4324/9781003635628-11

Together, these aims invite educators to reimagine what occupation-centered education can become and how it can shape the future of occupational therapy.

OBJECTIVES

This chapter will help educators to:

1. Summarize key principles and elements of occupation-centered education as guided by the SCIL-OT Model.
2. Recognize ways of using the SCIL-OT Model in conjunction with other approaches to curriculum and learning design that can enhance occupation-centered education.
3. Imagine new schema for organizing knowledge for occupation-centered education in occupational therapy.
4. Recall the significance of creating robust occupation-centered programs, courses, class sessions, practice education experiences, and assessment strategies.

SYNOPSIS

As elaborated throughout this book, the SCIL-OT Model outlines the essential elements of occupation-centered education. These elements include the core subject of occupation—the central concern that the profession exists to address through education, practice, and research. Additional elements include topics, knowledge communities, and the context of learning situations.

The SCIL-OT Model also provides a set of explicit principles and practical guidelines that educators can use to center both their teaching and students' learning. Among the most important are the following:

1. Occupation is the core subject of occupational therapy—and therefore the core subject of occupational therapy education.
2. Teaching occupation means teaching the dynamics of occupation as a mechanism of health and well-being and helping students understand how specific occupations activate those dynamics.
3. Topics are necessary and wide-ranging, but most are not inherently distinctive to occupational therapy. Their relevance emerges when they are intentionally connected to the core subject of occupation.
4. Students learn about occupation through engagement with diverse knowledge communities. These communities support students in becoming active knowledge developers and contributors within the profession.

5. Occupation-centered teaching and learning occur "on-the-lines" of the SCIL-OT Model. Educators must design learning experiences that prompt students to
   - connect topics to the core subject of occupation.
   - connect their own lives to the core subject of occupation.
   - connect topics to other topics—and collectively to occupation.
   - connect learning to diverse knowledge communities.

As the title of this book suggests, the SCIL-OT Model offers extensive guidance for designing occupation-centered curricula across four component areas: the education program, its courses, its class sessions, and its approaches to practice education.

At the same time, we believe educators can use the SCIL-OT Model in tandem with other curriculum design approaches that are not explicitly occupation-centered. In the next section, we explore how the SCIL-OT Model can complement two such approaches: Fink's (2013) backward learning design for academic courses and AOTA's (2021) Occupational Therapy Curriculum Design Framework for developing new occupational therapy curricula.

USING THE SCIL-OT MODEL TO AUGMENT OTHER APPROACHES TO CURRICULUM AND LEARNING DESIGN

In his book, *Creating Significant Learning Experiences: An Integrated Approach to Designing College Courses*, Fink (2013) details the use of backward design for developing academic courses across diverse disciplines. Backward design emphasizes a learning-centered approach, rather than a content-centered one. According to Fink, when educators adopt a content-centered approach, they often begin by listing the topics their course will cover. In contrast, a learning-centered approach begins with the end in mind. For example, an educator might ask: *What will students need to be able to do two years from now as a result of having taken this course?*

Thus, the backward in backward design refers to starting with situational analysis and desired learning outcomes, then working backward to select learning activities and content. We are proponents of backward design as described by Fink and have integrated its process with SCIL-OT principles to develop curricula across programs, courses, class sessions, and practice education.

The Occupational Therapy Curriculum Design Framework of AOTA (2021) offers educators a practical and detailed guide for designing occupational therapy and occupational therapy assistant curricula. This approach highlights key influential factors throughout the design process, including an institution's mission and context; opportunities for community partnerships; societal needs; current clinical practices and accreditation requirements; and student characteristics and expectations. We also support this framework's emphasis on interrelated factors and continuous curriculum improvement.

Although neither Fink's (2013) backward design nor AOTA's (2021) framework explicitly guides occupation-centered education, we believe their processes can effectively support it when used in conjunction with SCIL-OT principles. When considered through the lens of occupation-centered education, these design steps become more focused and targeted—helping educators center learning on occupation and its transformative potential.

RE-IMAGINING THE OCCUPATIONAL THERAPY CURRICULUM

The SCIL-OT Model is a valuable tool in supporting occupational therapy educators to develop and deliver occupation-centered educational programs. While many educational programs have embraced an occupation-centered approach to education already, the SCIL-OT Model is the first framework to provide tangible and practical support to novice and experienced educators alike to enhance the occupation focus of their programs and educational practice.

Ultimately, however, the SCIL-OT Model points toward something greater than the above principles and guidelines. The model points toward the possibility of reimaging how we organize knowledge through the occupational therapy curriculum.

Occupational therapy education programs organize knowledge in various ways.

1. Some programs organize knowledge by lifespan stages—children, adolescents, adults, and older adults. This schema shows students how practice is shaped by stages of the lifespan. It can overlook, however, what is the same about occupational therapy regardless of lifespan stage.
2. Some programs organize knowledge by subspecialties—physical disabilities, mental health, neurology, or orthotics, as examples. These can also be useful schema and yet they likely foreground knowledge of health conditions and body functions and structures as primary knowledge for occupational therapy.
3. Still another schema organizes knowledge by practice setting—hospitals, community, schools, for example. This schema is beneficial in supporting students' pragmatic reasoning about how the setting shapes practices. It, too, however, can miss what holds practice together across so many settings.

4. Some programs use the occupational therapy process to organize knowledge by creating courses on assessment and intervention. Spreading the occupational therapy process out across different semesters can make it challenging for students to piece together or to recognize that assessment and intervention are continuous and simultaneous, not distinct processes.

In our view, organizing knowledge according to the field's distinctive ideas and questions is an overlooked schema for programs, courses, class sessions, and practice experiences. We imagine the core of occupational therapy education becoming crystalized in a commitment that would reshape how we organize and construct curricula. For example, if adopted whole-heartedly, what effect might the following statement have on curriculum design?

> *The occupational therapy profession will define, promote, and educate novices about occupation as the foundation for optimizing the health and well-being of societies. Occupation is core knowledge for occupational therapy education, practice and research.*

Imagine how a commitment like this might modify what courses we create, what learning outcomes we select and deselect across the program, courses, classes, and practice education experiences; how we focus our assessments and learning activities; and what content we do and do not include.

Imagine what might ensue in our curricula and practice education experiences if we designed them from a perspective that the most fundamental thing to know is occupation as the most basic element for human health and well-being. Imagine what educational experiences might arise if a primary aim of education was to have students promote health in direct relation to occupational engagement and experience.

We imagine that no matter what our graduates may be helping clients with—a transfer, a splint, using the subway, making street art, life in a refugee camp—they would easily and continuously explain how that thing relates to occupational engagement broadly and how such engagement supports health and well-being. We imagine these conversations not as superficial statements like "this will support your health and well-being" but in knowledgeable, clear explanations of how occupation works in health and well-being, why it works, what consequences can arise without it. We imagine that conversation taking place with individual clients, their supporters, community leaders, and politicians.

THE SIGNIFICANCE OF RE-IMAGINING OCCUPATIONAL THERAPY EDUCATION

Therefore, the SCIL-OT model ultimately points beyond even occupational performance and participation as the core of occupational therapy. It leads us to grapple with why we care about performance and engagement at all, with why occupation is the most fundamental element of health and well-being, and with how to teach in ways that fulfill our societal contract to sustain that construct.

Continuing to grapple with these important concepts and their manifestation in how we select and organize knowledge through courses and teaching and learning experiences is critical to the fulfillment of occupational therapy's vision. Continuing to work out these concepts is also critical to the advancement of just and inclusive societies around the world. Why? Diversity, inclusion, and belonging, from an occupational perspective, refer in part to people being able to access and participate in the occupations that are socioculturally meaningful to them and to be free to perform the occupations in the ways and contexts they are accustomed.

Further, inclusion and belonging derive directly from being able to access and participate in the occupations of one's community. Inclusion and belonging, expressed through access and participation in occupation, are the basis for healthy individuals, communities, and populations.

Therefore, it behooves us to create education grounded in occupational justice wherein all occupational therapy students (1) appreciate that the ways people engage in occupation varies across diverse sociocultural contexts; (2) with cultural humility, seek to understand clients' unique history of doing things in particular ways; (3) uphold the rights of all people to engage in the occupations that are meaningful to them, in ways that are meaningful to them; and (4) work collaboratively to enable access to and participation in diverse occupations.

This work of realizing and strengthening occupation-centered education is a deeply felt professional calling. So it is that this work has deeply called to us. Just as this work calls, we believe, to innumerable other occupational therapy educators worldwide.

REFERENCES

American Occupational Therapy Association. (2021). Occupational therapy curriculum design framework. *American Journal of Occupational Therapy*, *75*(Suppl. 3), 751343001. https://doi.org/10.5014/ajot.2021.75S3008

Fink, L. D. (2013). *Creating significant learning experiences: An integrated approach to designing college courses*. Jossey-Bass.

Index

Note: Page numbers in *italics* indicate a figure and page numbers in **bold** indicate a table on the corresponding page.

For Product Safety Concerns and Information please contact our EU representative GPSR@taylorandfrancis.com
Taylor & Francis Verlag GmbH, Kaufingerstraße 24, 80331 München, Germany

www.ingramcontent.com/pod-product-compliance
Ingram Content Group UK Ltd.
Pitfield, Milton Keynes, MK11 3LW, UK
UKHW020005200926
475702UK00015B/2492
* 9 7 8 1 0 4 1 0 6 4 8 4 8 *